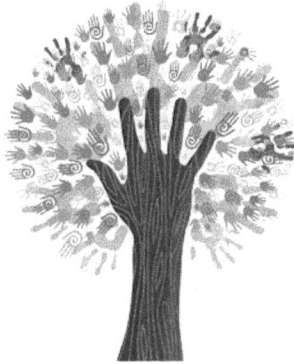

REACH CHRONICLES

A Community Mental Health Model for Children and Adolescents in Singapore

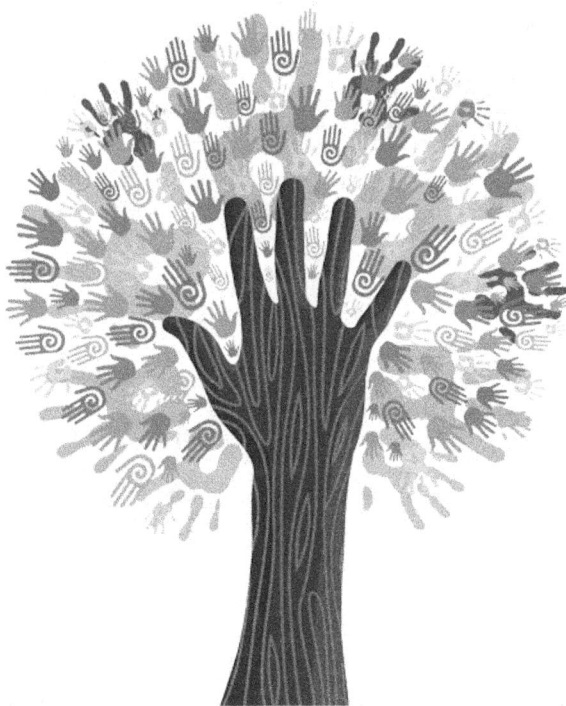

REACH CHRONICLES

REACCH CHRONICLES

A Community Mental Health Model for Children and Adolescents in Singapore

Editors

D. Fung, L. P. Ong, S. L. Tay & W. H. Sim

Institute of Mental Health, Singapore

World Scientific

NEW JERSEY · LONDON · SINGAPORE · BEIJING · SHANGHAI · HONG KONG · TAIPEI · CHENNAI

Published by

World Scientific Publishing Co. Pte. Ltd.

5 Toh Tuck Link, Singapore 596224

USA office: 27 Warren Street, Suite 401-402, Hackensack, NJ 07601

UK office: 57 Shelton Street, Covent Garden, London WC2H 9HE

British Library Cataloguing-in-Publication Data
A catalogue record for this book is available from the British Library.

REACH CHRONICLES
A Community Mental Health Model for Children and Adolescents in Singapore

ISBN 978-981-4440-36-3 (pbk)

Typeset by Stallion Press
EmaiL: enquiries@stallionpress.com

Printed in Singapore by Mainland Press Pte Ltd.

Contents

Foreword

Chua Hong Choon
CEO, Institute of Mental Health

This is a book about the journey undertaken by REACH, the first community mental healthcare programme for children and adolescents in Singapore. Readers will be able to see the development of innovative services in our mental healthcare through the lenses of professionals from various disciplines. The book also describes the strengthening of partnerships among the educational, mental health and social services sectors, with the common goal of creating more effective intervention pathways for young people with mental health problems.

The public health framework that underpins this book reminds us that the objective of any intervention — whether school-, family-, or community-based is to halt the progression of mental health problems in young people through a combination of efforts. This book aims to generate more dialogues within and across school and healthcare communities that can lead to the enhancement of mental health services.

As the REACH project matures into its fifth year of implementation, it is fitting that we celebrate our achievements and successes. Appreciation goes to the REACH team — their dedication and commitment have paved the way for this book, which documents how we have arrived at this major milestone towards community mental healthcare for children and adolescents.

Preface

Daniel Fung
REACH Programme Director

There is a Nigerian saying — "it takes a whole village to raise a child". It helps us to understand why, when it comes to helping children, the efforts of everyone in the community is required.

Our team at the Department of Child and Adolescent Psychiatry started life as a part-time clinic in 1970 with a mandate common for child guidance clinics in various parts of the world, i.e. to educate the mind, protect the body (of the child as in preventing abuse) and punish the offender. Over time, the Child Guidance Clinics of the Institute of Mental Health did that but with an underlying focus on treating mental health disorders and more importantly, preventing them. This search for a preventative approach led our teams to work closely with schools and other community agencies. Child mental health professionals led by psychiatrists started to look beyond the scope of mental health, and spend more time outside the clinic and hospital. We would spend much of our time initially in primary medical care settings like polyclinics, and eventually to the community where children congregate, and the schools.

REACH was the culmination of a year of discussions with professionals in child mental health. From pioneer developmental paediatricians like Professor Ho Lai Yun and Specialist Educational experts like Dr Mariam Aljunied, it was evident that a school-based network not only provides early intervention but can prevent the need to seek help in a tertiary clinical service. In the last ten years, "our village" has developed the concept of a comprehensive child and youth mental health service that is not hospital-centric but community-centric.

The REACH Chronicles marks the beginning of our journey. As a village, REACH will continue to learn and grow in hope that the lessons learnt will propel us to the next frontier. These are the voyages of the work of our village, the chronicles of REACH.

Acknowledgement

In the production of the REACH Chronicles, many parties came together to bring it to fruition. Its success is as much the efforts of the authors, editors and the many advisors and reviewers; as well as our partners, whether singly or as organisations.

We would like to thank the medical professionals who were generous in providing the framework of our work. We would like to thank Dr Cai Yiming, whose steadfastness saw the discipline of child psychiatry grow within Singapore and beyond. With the support of Dr Ong Say How, Dr Helen Chen, Dr John Wong (Heads of Departments of Department of Child & Adolescent Psychiatry, IMH, Department of Psychological Medicine in KKH and NUH respectively), the REACH team members involved in the workgroup were given the autonomy to develop the book from concept to the final product. The workgroup is represented by all the four REACH teams: Ms Sim Wan Hua and Dr Wong Hui Yi (North), Ms July Lies (South), Mr Brian Poh (East 2010/11), Ms Estelle Lim (East), Ms Haslinda Ibrahim and Ms Cheryl KY Lee (West team).

Special thanks to Ms Tay So Leng as the workgroup head, who spent many tireless hours with Ms Han Bing Ling, administrative lead, to spearhead, guide and ensure content and professional administrative structures be put in place for this complex task of writing a book. The editing experience of this book also reflects the over-arching philosophy of the REACH community mental health project where efforts and responses of many people and organisations matter. For this, we want to acknowledge the Ministry of Education, Ministry of Health, National Council of Social Services and team leaders of REACH North, South, East, and West (Ms Geraldine Wong, Mr Ong Lue Ping, Ms Jocelyn Neo, Dr Delphine Koh, Ms Haslinda Ibrahim). In addition, we also highly value the inputs from Ms Chan Mei Chern, Assistant Director of Patient Operations and Ms Ting Mei See, Director of Corporate Communications of IMH. We are also extremely grateful for the editorial inputs by Dr Helen Chen (Head of Mental Wellness Service, KKH), Ms Ichha Oberoi (Manager, Corporate Communications, KKH) and Ms Goh Sze Ling (Corporate Communications, NUH). Appreciation also goes to Ms Winnie Koh and Ms Christine Tan for their editing advice.

We would also like to express our gratitude to our partners in the publication of the REACH Chronicles: our photographer, Haanusia Prithivi Raj, and the children who contributed their drawings. In addition, Ms Shirley Chen (Personal Assistant to Dr Fung), school counsellors, educators, GPs, social workers, parents and students — although we are unable to name everyone, we are grateful to all who have extended the network of community mental health services for the good of the students in Singapore. For the children and families that we have interacted with, the examples that we have used are composite histories and real names have not been used.

It has been a fulfilling journey and the REACH team looks forward to constantly innovating and improving the state of mental healthcare delivery in Singapore.

Contributors to the REACH Chronicles: Authors & Editors

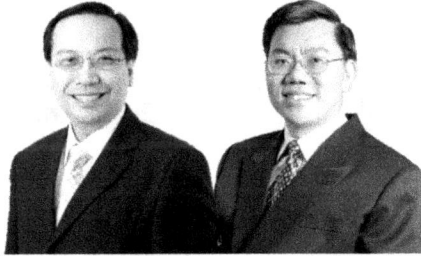

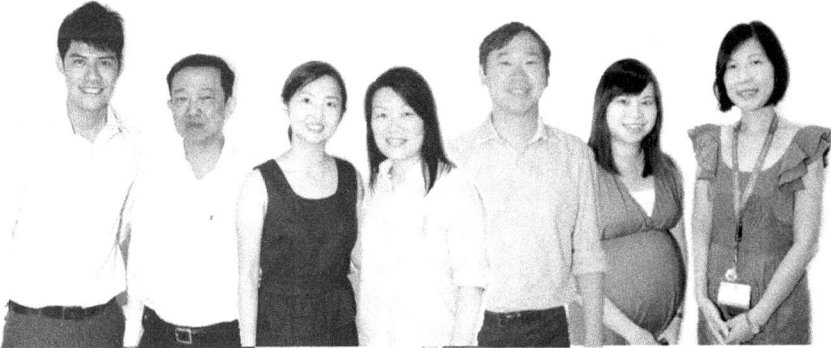

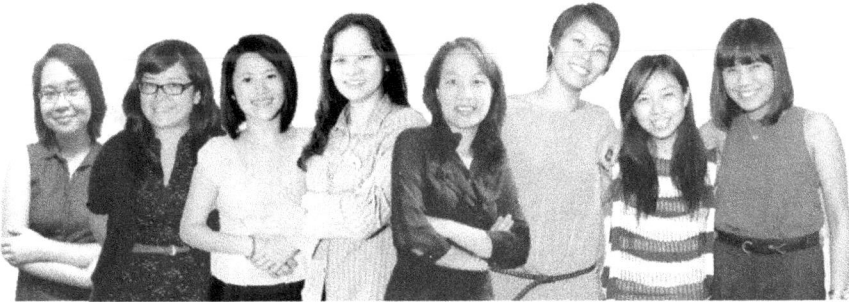

Top row from left: Associate Professor Daniel Fung, Professor John Wong.
Second row from left: Poh Zhi Qian Brian, Dr Cai Yiming, Sim Wan Hua, Tay So Leng, Ong Lue Ping, Han Bing Ling, Chan Mei Chern.
Bottom row from left: Cheryl Lee, Dr Wong Hui Yi, July Lies, Liew Shiang Hui, Estelle Lim, Dr Delphine Koh, Cheak Ching Cheng, Jillian Boon.

Introduction

Brian Poh and Cai Yiming

The meaning of REACH

REACH
Pronunciation:/rēCH/
verb

- stretch out an arm in a specified direction in order to touch or grasp something
- (reach out) extend help, understanding, or influence: *he felt such an urge to reach out to his fellow sufferer*

(Oxford Dictionaries, 2012)

The REACH for Students project initiated in 2007 has stayed true to its namesake. According to Oxford Dictionaries (2012), to 'reach' is to stretch out an arm in a specified direction in order to touch or grasp something, and to 'reach out', is to extend help, understanding, or influence. Since its inception, REACH has sought to stretch out its arm, its helping arm, to extend help, understanding, and influence positively, our mental health at-risk children and adolescents in the community.

REACH is a community-based mental health service in Singapore, set up to support schools, community agencies and family doctors helping children and adolescents with emotional, behavioural or neuro-developmental issues. The name 'REACH' is an acronym for **R**esponse,

Early intervention, Assessment for Community mental Health. Response, as the first word of the acronym, is what REACH does fundamentally- to Respond to children and adolescents with mental, emotional or behavioural difficulties. This response constitutes many different components such as answering queries from counsellors, accepting referrals, and more importantly, providing Early intervention and Assessment for students. The last two letters of the acronym sums up the context of REACH's service: Community-based, as opposed to a clinical setting; and its focus on the mental Health issues of children and adolescents in Singapore.

The birth of REACH

There were several key contexts that highlighted the need for a service in Singapore that caters to the young population with mental illness. These were the basis for why REACH was formed. Three main contexts are imperative in the understanding of REACH's origins: the background of mental illness, particularly with regards to children and adolescents in Singapore, the existing services for children and adolescents in Singapore prior to REACH and the National Mental Health Blueprint which REACH is a part of. The background of mental illness gives readers a clearer picture of the prevalence and impact of mental illness around the world, and particularly the children and adolescent population in Singapore. This emphasised the enormity of the need for a service that caters to the young population in Singapore with mental illness. A look at the existing services for children and adolescents in Singapore gives the reader an evolutionary run-through of how REACH was conceived. Finally, we will give the readers some key information on the national mental health policy from which REACH is conceptualised.

The burden of mental illness

Epidemiology of mental illness around the world

Mental illness is very pervasive in the world today. This is evident from the latest World Mental Health (WMH) Surveys conducted by the World

Health Organization (WHO), where large-scale data was collected from over 85,000 respondents worldwide, covering seventeen countries in Africa, Asia, the Americas, Europe, and the Middle East (Kessler *et al.*, 2007b). The psychiatric diagnoses in the WMH Surveys are based on the Composite International Diagnostic Interview (CIDI) developed by the WHO (Kessler & Ustun, 2004), which generates four core DSM-IV diagnoses of anxiety disorders, mood disorders, impulse control disorders and substance use disorders (American Psychiatric Association, 2000).

The results are staggering, with the estimated lifetime prevalence of having one or more of the mental disorders ranging from 12.0% in Nigeria to 47.4% in the United States. The inter-quartile range (IQR; 25th–75th percentiles) of this estimated lifetime prevalence across the seventeen countries is 18.1% to 36.1%. Both anxiety disorders and mood disorders are highly prevalent, with lifetime prevalence of the former ranging from 4.8% to 31.0% (IQR: 9.9–16.7%) and the latter ranging from 3.3% to 21.4% (IQR: 9.8–15.8%).

In a comparative study of the prevalence of mental illness and other major diseases, the report on the 'Global Burden of Disease' by WHO (2008) showed that worldwide, the prevalence of unipolar depressive disorders (151.2 million) is higher than tuberculosis (13.9 million) and HIV infection (31.4 million) combined. The figures for bipolar affective disorders and schizophrenia stand at 29.5 million and 26.3 million respectively. No statistics are available for anxiety disorders, which are even more prevalent than mood disorders as shown by the WMH Surveys. If a hypothetical figure is to be calculated for the combined prevalence of all mental illness, it could possibly be higher than the prevalence for diabetes mellitus (220.5 million), one of the leading causes of deaths in the world (WHO, 2008).

A pragmatic and standardised metric to study the impact of diseases is the disability-adjusted life year (DALY), which represents the lost year of 'healthy' life by being in states of poor health or disability (Murray, 1996). The DALY takes into account both the number of years of life lost (YLL) from premature mortality and years of life lived in less than full health (years of life lost through disability; YLD). The DALY gives a good comparison and macro perspective of the impact of different illness, through the measure of years of life lost from death and disability. While none of the mental disorders are in the top ten of the 'leading causes of death', unipolar depressive disorder, bipolar disorder and schizophrenia are among the leading global causes of YLD, with unipolar depressive disorders being the leader causing 65.3 million years of life lost globally (WHO, 2008). Even though the direct mortality of mental illness is low, the amount of disability that it causes is a considerable burden to healthcare. In fact, unipolar depressive disorder is the third leading burden of disease worldwide, as calculated using DALYs. 65.5 million DALYs are lost from unipolar depressive disorder, compared to 58.5 million DALYs from acquired immune deficiency syndrome (AIDS), 46.6 million DALYs from "cerebrovascular" disease and 19.7 DALYs from diabetes mellitus (WHO, 2008). Given the global prevalence and substantial negative impact of mental illness, it is thus necessary that at a local level, Singapore addresses mental health issues in its healthcare services and policies.

Epidemiology of mental illness in Singapore

The worrying worldwide statistics of mental illness gives an indication of the situation in Singapore. In the mid-1990s, a mental health survey was conducted on 3,020 citizens to study the epidemiology of psychiatric morbidity of the general population (Fones, Kua, Ng, & Ko, 1998). Using the CIDI (the same diagnostic instrument used in the WMH Surveys) and the General Health Questionnaire, the participants were interviewed to detect any minor psychiatric disturbances corresponding to the International Classification of Diseases (ICD-10) criteria (WHO, 1992). The results showed that one in six Singaporeans are believed to suffer from mental illness. According to The Singapore Burden of Disease 2004, anxiety and depression accounted for nearly 11.8% of the overall YLD burden in Singapore (Phua, Chua, Ma, Heng, & Chew, 2009). As the total number of years of "healthy" life lost as a result of disability was 188,701 years, this means that over 22,000 "healthy" years were lost as a result of anxiety and depression. With such a high prevalence rate and accountability for ill-health, it is a pressing issue for mental health policy-makers to effectively respond to these individuals with mental illness (Fones *et al.*, 1998).

A more recent Singapore Mental Health Study spearheaded by the Institute of Mental Health (IMH) was conducted in 2010 to examine the prevalence of common mental illness in the adult Singapore resident population (National Healthcare Group, 2011). The survey showed that depression has affected over 60,000 adult men and 110,000 adult women during their lifetime in Singapore, while some 100,000 people have suffered from anxiety disorders during their lifetime. Although these figures appear more optimistic compared to those in other developed countries (Kessler *et al.*, 2007a), it is anticipated that the strains on the mental wellbeing of Singaporeans will grow, as the population ages, family sizes shrink and accompanied economic burdens increase (Ministry of Health, 2007).

Mental illness in Singapore's children and adolescents

There is much knowledge gleaned from these statistics of adult population that can be translated to the younger population in Singapore. It is important to remember that all adults were once children and adolescents and not to treat them as different beings. Moreover, some of the mental illness that hit the adults might have begun when they were children or adolescents. A review of recent literature on the age of onset of mental disorders (Kessler *et al.*, 2007b) based on the WHO World Mental Health surveys, found that the onset of mental disorders usually occurs in childhood or adolescence. In fact, approximately half of all lifetime mental disorders in most studies start by mid-teens. Notably, the impulse-control disorders have the earliest age of onset distributions, with median age of onset across countries at 7 to 9 years for attention-deficit/hyperactivity disorder (ADHD), 7 to 15 years for oppositional-defiant disorder (ODD) and 9 to 14 years for conduct disorder (CD). 80% of all lifetime ADHD are diagnosed in the age range 4 to 11 years, while the vast majority of ODD and CD begins between ages 5 and 15 years. The study also showed that some anxiety disorders such as phobias and separation anxiety disorder (SAD)

Some Mental Disorders with Early Age of Onset

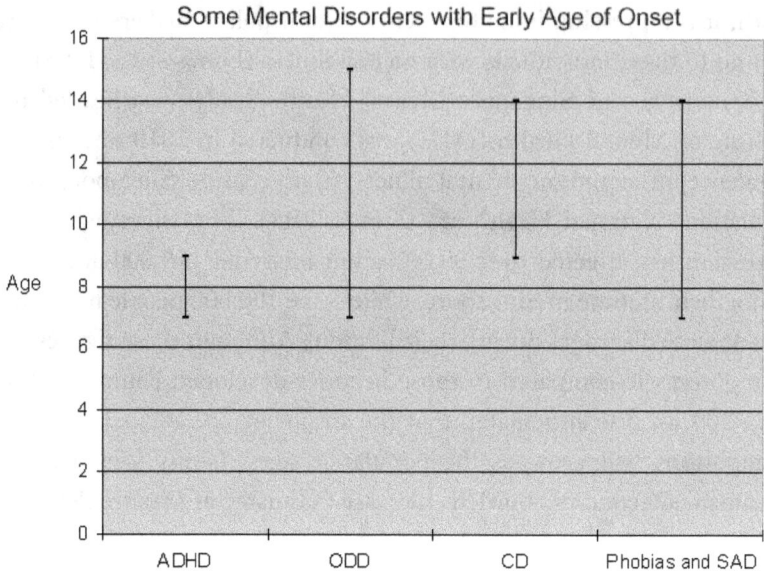

have very early age of onset distributions, with the median age of onset in the range of 7 to 14 years.

Besides learning that half of all lifetime mental disorders occur by mid-teens and some mental disorders start at childhood and adolescence, Christiana, Gilman, Guardino, Mickelson , Morselli , Olfson and Kessler (2000) also found that people tend to delay more than a decade after the first onset of a mental disorder before seeking treatment. By then, these individuals often have other highly co-morbid conditions that would have been more treatable if they had sought help earlier. Various studies have shown that early intervention provides improvements and better prognosis of the symptoms of anxiety disorders (Dadds, Holland, Laurens, Mullins, Barrett & Spence, 1999; Hirshfeld-Becker & Biederman, 2002), mood disorders (Harrington & Clark, 1998; Petersen, Compas, Brooks-Gunn, Stemmler & Grant, 1993) and impulse control disorders such as ADHD (Rappaport, Ornoy, & Tenenbaum, 1998) and conduct disorders (Kaiser & Hester, 1997). Early intervention in children and adolescents in Singapore thus mitigates the course of these often debilitating disorders.

In addition to the poorer prognosis of psychiatric disorders in adulthood, there are also proximate consequences of untreated mental disorders in children and adolescents. Psychotic disorder, depression and conduct disorder have been identified as risk factors in adolescent suicide (Cai, 1998). According to the Samaritans of Singapore, the suicide rate among youth aged 12 to 19 hit a five-year high in 2009 (Hoe, 2010). The rates of teenage suicides was 19 in the year 2009, up from 12 cases in year 2008, amounting to an increase of almost 60% (Samaritans of Singapore, 2010). School failure is also highly correlated with mental disorders in youth. According to data from the United States, about 50% of students with mental illness drop out of high school, making it the highest dropout rate of any disability group (U.S. Department of Education, 2001). Mental health disorders are also implicated in juvenile delinquency and incarceration of adolescents (Cocozza & Skowyra, 2000; Grisso, 1999; Robertson, Dill, Husain & Undesser, 2004).

The Singapore Mental Health Study done on the Singaporean adult populations showed that many adult mental health disorders had onset in childhood and adolescence. In 2003, Woo *et al.* (2007) from the Department of Child and Adolescent Psychiatry of the Institute of Mental Health completed a study to determine the prevalence of emotional and behavioural issues in a large community sample of Singapore children aged 6 to 12 years old. The results show that based on the Child Behaviour Checklist (CBCL), 12.5% of the sample have either emotional or behavioural problems. A further breakdown of the problems reveals that 12.2% have internalising problems such as withdrawn behaviour, somatic complaints, anxiety and depression, while 4.9% have externalising problems such as aggressive and delinquent behaviour. This is comparable to the statistics in the West (Barkmann & Schulte-Markwort, 2005; Sawyer *et al.*, 2001) and India (Srinath, Girimaji, Gururaj, Seshadri, Subbakrishna, Bhola & Kumar, 2005) but higher than China (Liu, Kurita, Guo, Miyake, Ze & Cao, 1999). In essence, a good mental healthcare service for children and adolescents is not only beneficial, but essential for the mental health of the nation. Singapore has recognised this since late the 1960s, which led to the establishment of child psychiatry in the then Woodbridge Hospital.

Child and Adolescent Psychiatry in Singapore

Singapore's healthcare system and tertiary psychiatric hospital

According to Tucci (2004) in a global healthcare market review, Singapore has "one of the most successful healthcare systems in the world, in terms of both efficiency in financing and the results achieved in community health outcomes". Good and affordable healthcare is available to all Singaporeans through subsidised medical services at public hospitals and clinics. The philosophy of individual responsibility towards health is promoted through the 'co-payment' of medical expenses, with the support of Medisave (a compulsory medical savings scheme) and Medishield (national insurance scheme) schemes. For those who cannot afford the heavily subsidised bill charges, an endowment fund known as Medifund is available as a 'safety net' (Ministry of Health, 2012). The '3M' framework of Medisave, Medishield and Medifund effectively ensures that the individual makes a significant contribution to his or her own healthcare costs, and allows the government to maintain a relatively trim spending on the public health system. Currently, Singapore spends about 4.0% of its GDP on healthcare (Ministry of Health, 2011).

IMH serves as the main psychiatric arm of Singapore's Healthcare System. IMH started out as a 30-bed building in 1841, dejectedly called 'The Insane Hospital' (Ng, 2001). Since then, huge advances have been made in terms of treatment, training and research. IMH is now a 2,000-bed acute tertiary psychiatric hospital situated on a 25-hectare campus at Buangkok Green Medical Park, with modern facilities and multi-discipline departments to provide holistic care for the patients. IMH is the first mental health institution in Asia to receive the Joint Commission International (JCI) Accreditation in 2005. In 2011, IMH clinched the inaugural Grand Award for the Hospital of the Year, a Winner award and two Excellence awards at the Asian Hospital Management Awards, which recognise and honour hospitals in Asia that carry out best practices.

1968 early semblance to child and adolescent psychiatry

The early semblance to Child and Adolescent Psychiatry was first provided from 1968 to 69 by a psychiatrist and a psychologist at Woodbridge Hospital (now IMH/Woodbridge Hospital). It was actually more of a programme of mutual referrals rather than the traditional child guidance team approach. There were no specialist personnel or facilities to treat emotional and behavioural disorders in children and adolescents. Inevitably, some of the more seriously disturbed children and adolescents had to be admitted to the adult wards of Woodbridge Hospital.

In January 1970, the Minster of Health, in his address at a regional workshop for mental health, announced the government's intention to develop child guidance clinics. This was a significant move in our mental health services.

1970 Child Guidance Clinic

On the 7th of April 1970, the Ministry of Health established a Child Guidance Clinic (CGC) to cater to the needs of children and adolescents with psychological and emotional disorders. It started as a part-time child guidance clinic which operated out of an old bungalow on the grounds of the Outram Road General Hospital (now known as Singapore General Hospital). The clinic was staffed by a psychiatrist, psychologist, social worker and a nurse and operated on an equivalent of two full days a week.

However, in mid-January 1971, the roof collapsed and the building had to be abandoned after it was declared unfit for occupation. The clinic was moved to old Kallang Airport Road and assumed service on 17th of March 1971 on a three days per week basis. The staff strength grew to include a medical officer and another social worker. CGC remained at the Kallang Maternal and Child Health Clinic for two years. By 1972, it was operating full time to meet the growing need for more care of the young, which still holds true to this day.

"In Singapore, we have a young population. More than half of the population is under the age of 21 years. It is therefore important that we should lay sufficient emphasis on the provisions of adequate medical services for the young, who form so large a segment of our population. As a nation, it is worthwhile investment for Singapore to start thinking seriously of such provisions as Well Child Clinics and Adolescent Clinics. It is, to my mind, far better if they are seen at regular intervals even if apparently healthy — to make sure that they are developing sound minds in healthy bodies" (Phoon, 1972).

The clinic at Outram Road General Hospital was soon relocated to the pre-war nurses' hostel (annexe building), Russels Road, at Alexandra Park. Dr Wong Sze Tai headed the clinic. Facilities were limited but the mood was one of hope amidst great struggling.

"The place is hardly inviting and not one which children would look forward to visiting weekly or even fortnightly. In fact, because of its lack of facilities, like a small canteen or a more cheerful waiting area, parents are often seen dozing off on the old chairs as their children are undergoing guidance sessions" (The Straits Times, 1979, June).

Thus in 1980, the clinic moved to a more convenient and better-equipped facility at the Institute of Health in Outram Road. In the same year, Dr Goh Choo Woon went to London on a Loke's scholarship for a year's specialist training in family therapy at the Hospital for Sick Children at Great Ormond Street. It was under his leadership that the practice of family therapy became widely used at the clinic.

Modern technology was used to teach proper interview and counselling skills at the clinic. An interview room was converted into a soundproof recording studio separated by a one-way mirror from an adjourning observation room. Medical students, psychologists and other doctors would use the observation room to watch, through the one way mirror; family interview or therapy sessions, which could be simultaneously recorded on video for further demonstration and evaluation. This method is an effective way of teaching proper interview and counselling skills and is widely used in the west.

Video-recordings of doctors' sessions with children were made under the written consent of the parents. With the tapes, doctors were able to make more detailed analysis and seek a second opinion if there were diagnostic problems. Sometimes, the behaviour tells the real story, like a stare from the parent to silence a child. With videotapes, you can freeze the action, replay and re-examine a point.

1982 Child and Adolescent Inpatient Unit

In 1982, an 18-bed Child and Adolescent Inpatient Unit, converted from the old matron's quarter, was opened at Woodbridge Hospital for the management of older children and adolescents with disturbed emotion and behaviours.

Children who present problems in diagnosis may require systematic observation and investigation as short-term inpatients, which may range from two weeks to three months. This step is needed to exclude home influences in a clinical problem. During the inpatient period, the child's parents will meet the staff to clarify issues. All these are done so that the child can be discharged eventually to a home that has improved so much that it is suitable for the patient.

A few factors that determine whether it is necessary to admit a child for inpatient treatment are the severity of the problem, the safety of the child (for example in highly suicidal teenagers), the lack of response to outpatient treatment and the complexity of the family problem.

The most common conditions that require admission for inpatient treatment include suicidal behaviour, psychotic conditions, conduct disorder, anorexia nervosa, persistent school refusal, aggressive and violent behaviour. The admission allows close observation, longer duration of treatments as well as relief from strained relationships.

In 2005, the in-patient unit was revamped and renovated to keep the patients in graded levels of care so that the most disturbed patients were kept in the secure and low stimulation end of the ward while the recovered patients were allowed to move freely in the outer-most part of the ward and patients in different stages of recovery took up the middle portion of the ward. There was ample space for sports and recreational activities for the patients and a cosy visitors' room for parents and other family members. The in-patient ward was also re-named the Sunrise Wing under the umbrella of the CGC.

For security and legal reasons, young offenders admitted under the Children and Young Persons Act 1993, were sent to the adult forensic unit of Woodbridge Hospital. They could also be remanded at the Singapore Boys' Home, Toa Payoh Girls' Home or the Changi Medical Complex for psychiatric evaluation.

1993 Department of Child and Adolescent Psychiatry

In April 1993, the Department of Child and Adolescent Psychiatry was formed at the opening of the new and modern Institute of Mental Health/ Woodbridge Hospital at Buangkok Green Medical Park in Hougang. The department was headed by Dr Cai Yiming.

In June 1993, the Smoking Cessation Clinic at the Child Guidance Clinic was started in response to the upsurge in smoking among the youths in Singapore and a law which banned smoking among children and adolescents under the age of 18.

The Smoking Cessation Clinic provided assessment, counselling and group workshop programmes using mainly a psychological and behavioural approach to about 500 to 600 new smokers a year. They were referred to the clinic by school teachers (about 93%), parents or health enforcement officers (7%) who caught them smoking. At the completion of the programmes, about 20% of the adolescents quit smoking completely, with the rest showing a reduction of about 50% in the average number of cigarettes smoked a day.

1998 Publication of Book on "Help Your Child to Cope"

In 1998, Dr Cai Yiming and Dr Daniel Fung from IMH wrote a book, "Help Your Child To Cope-Understanding Childhood Stress". This is a book on children who need to cope with a large amount of stress in Singapore. The response to this first book was surprisingly good. The book was subsequently translated into a Chinese edition the next year. As a result, they were encouraged to produce a second book, "Raise Your Child Right — A Parenting Guide For The 0–6 Years Old", in 2002. It highlights the essential principles of bringing up children in the tender years, which are the critical formative years before they enter formal schooling. Dr Fung and Dr Rebecca Ang also wrote a book on dealing with angry children, often one of the most difficult aspects of parenting. This book is aptly titled as "Seeing Red". Knowing how marital conflicts in parents have a significant impact on the mental health of the children, Dr Cai wrote "When Parents Fight, The Children Cry!" to explain and provide advice on the issues of custody and access, ramifications of divorce and the effect of divorce on parents, as well as children. In 2008, an important volume "A Primer of Child and Adolescent Psychiatry" written by members of the Child and Adolescent Psychiatry Department of IMH, and edited by Dr Fung and Dr Cai, was published. The multi-disciplinary team members in the department also produced a series of 12 books on the different mental health issues for children. These books chronicle the combined experiences of the multidisciplinary team, (including doctors, nurses, psychologists, social workers and occupational therapists) on the clinical practice of child and adolescent psychiatry.

With the appointment of Prof Gordon Parker as the Director of Research at the Institute of Mental Health, more clinical research on child and adolescent psychiatry were conducted. Public forums and media interviews on child and adolescent mental health issues were also actively pursued in the past few years. Parent support groups for ADHD and eating disorders were also formed.

1998 was also an important milestone as the Child Guidance Clinic shifted to the modern and fully air-conditioned new premises at the Health Promotion Board (HPB) building in the Singapore General Hospital compound.

2002 Singapore International Foundation's Sponsorship to Cambodia

In 2002, the department responded to the request of the Singapore International Foundation to send a psychiatric team to Cambodia. The aim was to assist and share knowledge with colleagues in Cambodia on how to promote public education effectively on the various mental health issues that had affected the children of the country as a result of the internal social and political upheavals.

2004 Children's One-Stop Psycho-Educational Service (COPES)

In 2004, the department started to provide inputs to the Paediatric Department of the National University Hospital with the setting up of a Child Guidance Clinic. Another important milestone is the setting up of the COPES (Children's One-Stop Psycho-Educational Services) Programme to address the learning difficulties of children. This Health Service Development Project comprised comprehensive evaluation and intervention by a team of educational psychologists, specialist teachers, occupational therapists and speech therapists, under the direction of Dr Daniel Fung.

In addition to the services provided by the department, children and adolescents who required psychiatric assessment and treatment could also seek help at the private specialist's clinics and KK Women's and Children's Hospital.

2005 National Mental Health Blueprint

In 2005, with the increasing appreciation of mental health as a fundamental and crucial component of a person's well-being, the Ministry of Health appointed a committee of policy-makers and mental health professionals to formulate the first ever National Mental Health Blueprint for the years 2007 to 2012 (Ministry of Health, 2010). This is a great milestone in mental health service in Singapore and is also the policy from which REACH is born.

National Mental Health Blueprint

*Mental health is a fundamental and indispensable component of an individu-
al's health and well-being. Yet, mental illness is often neglected due to a lack*

of understanding, misconceptions, discrimination and stigma of the disease. Mental illness constitutes a significant burden of disease and adversely impacts on individuals, their families and society in terms of quality of life and financial costs. Across the world, there has been an increasing recognition of this enormous burden and it is timely to establish specific policies, plans and initiatives in Singapore to promote mental health and improve access to services.

(Prof K Satku, Director of Medical Services,
Ministry of Health, Foreword to
Healthy Minds, Healthy Communities 2010)

As Singapore progresses as a nation, social changes such as increasing divorce rates, family issues, work strains, academic stress and economic pressure pose mental health challenges for its people. A review of the National Mental Health Survey (Chua, Lim, Ng, Lee, Mahendran & Fones, 2004) found that the prevalence of mental disorders in Singapore is comparable to those of developing countries. This prompted the appointment of a committee in 2005. The role of this committee, consisting of policy-makers and mental health professionals from MOH, IMH, Health Promotion Board, various Restructured Hospitals, Ministry of Education (MOE) and the Ministry of Community Development, Youth and Sports (MCYS) was to formulate a new national mental health policy, named the National Mental Health Blueprint.

The Blueprint aims to promote mental health, prevent the development of mental health issues and reduce the impact of mental disorders. Its vision is to develop an emotionally resilient and mentally healthy community that has access to community-based, comprehensive and cost-effective mental health services.

The Blueprint is underpinned by eight key values:

1. Mental health encompasses both mental well-being and the absence of mental disorders;
2. Mental health is an integral part of general health;
3. Mental health promotion and care must be evidence-based and cost-effective;

4. Those with mental disorders should preferably be given appropriate services within the community;
5. Services should be accessible to everyone;
6. The mentally ill should not be discriminated against;
7. The needs and views of the mentally ill should be considered when planning, delivering and evaluating services;
8. Mental health care and promotion is a multi-sectoral effort.

In support of the Blueprint, the government announced in 2007 that it would invest S$88 million for this initiative from 2007 to 2011. In 2009, an additional S$35 million was injected to support the Blueprint (Ministry of Health, 2010).

In recognition that mental health issue is not just a medical problem but is affected by social factors (Engel, 1980), the Blueprint pushes for the move from a largely acute illness centred, hospital-based healthcare delivery system towards a community-based model of psychiatric care. A community-based service not only improves accessibility to services, but also reduces the stigma associated with mental illness (Burns, 2004). School personnel, general practitioners and family service centres are usually the first to observe early warning signs of mental health issues, and it is imperative that such community resources be tapped on to improve our mental health needs. The Blueprint also advocates the right-siting of care, where services are dispensed at the appropriate site, which may not always be in the hospital. This is especially so for milder cases, where intervention in the community is better for the patient as it reduces stigma and frees up scarce hospital beds for the more severe cases. Part of the Blueprint's plan to move towards community based psychiatric care is to form multidisciplinary community mental health teams for respective demographic and target groups in Singapore. They include Community Mental Health Team (CMHT) for adults, Aged Psychiatry Community Assessment & Treatment Service (APCATS) for the elderly and REACH for children and adolescents.

It was against such a backdrop that REACH was engendered. It took flight as a vision, in 2007, to stretch out its arm to extend help, understanding, and influence positively, our mental health at-risk children and adolescents in the community. Five years into its inception, it is timely to chronicle the journey of REACH and allow those within and outside the REACH network, to understand and appreciate the evolution and growth of REACH. The remaining chapters of this book detail this journey. We start with the Vision that started REACH in Chapter 1, with explanation of the population-based model of care and the REACH model. In Chapter 2, we look at the processes of REACH, from the initial referral to the assessment and finally management and intervention. In Chapter 3, we learn about the educational landscape of the schools in Singapore, both mainstream and in special education, as well as how REACH supports them. Chapter 4 explains and illustrates the partnering of REACH with Voluntary Welfare Organisations in Singapore, while Chapter 5 talks about the collaborations with general practitioners. The various resources utilised by REACH, including cognitive behavioural therapy programmes, groups, camps and research studies are listed in detail in Chapter 6. Last but not least, REACH's milestones and future directions are paved out in Chapter 7. Hopefully, this book will reach out to you and enable us to share REACH's ins and outs, ups and downs, and what holds for REACH in years to come. Read on, and enjoy the enREACHing journey ahead!

> *"Glory lies in the attempt to reach one's goal and not in reaching it"*
> Mahatma Gandhi

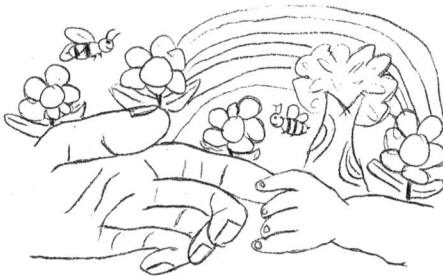

Chapter 1

The Vision

*Tay So Leng, Chan Mei Chern
and Daniel Fung*

A population-based model of care

An empirically-based philosophy towards the care of the mental health of our young was the underlying strategy when the mental health blueprint was initiated. In 1995, World Health Organisation (WHO) promoted the idea of health-promoting schools which showed that schools have a vital role in health risk amelioration (WHO, 1995). There have been a number of models of care which take a school-based approach towards mental health. The most convincing was a whole-of-school approach towards social and emotional learning in Sydney called the Gatehouse project (Bond, Patton, Glover, Carlin, Butler, Thomas & Bowes, 2004). In this project, 26 schools in several districts in Sydney participated in a randomised trial which showed that for over 3200 students, a multilevel intervention programme made significant headways in improving the mental health of the school population. This was evidence that a community-based intervention was effective in mental health promotion, and that such systems are complex and require sufficient funding and cooperation for it to be successful.

Our traditional model of care for child and adolescent psychiatry is one which is largely based on outpatient services with a small inpatient residential unit to treat severe cases. It is dependent on a referral system and assumes that children and adolescents with problems would be brought forward to utilise mental healthcare services. There is a discrepancy between cases presenting to clinics and actual prevalence data on mental health conditions which is termed as a treatment gap. In Singapore, we see an average of 3000 new referrals largely from schools and doctors, yet a local prevalence study in 2004 (Woo, Ng, Fung, Chan, Lee, Koh & Cai, 2007) showed that we may have about 50,000 (12.5% of the child population) children with mental health disorders in the community. This represents the treatment gap. In fact WHO has identified that the mental health gap is one of the major challenges in the future (WHO, 1995).

Clinic-based standardised care is the mainstay for treatment as it leverages on economies of scale. As awareness of mental health increases in the population, there is a challenge to meet the needs as referrals increase. In Singapore, this exponential growth in clinic referrals led to massive expansion of our services from attending to about 150 referrals in the first year of operation in 1970 to the more than 3000 referrals that we receive annually today. To meet this increase in demand, the Department of Child and Adolescent Psychiatry of the Institute of Mental (IMH) has expanded from two psychiatrists to a staff strength of more than 150 comprising doctors and various allied health professionals. However, due to the intensity of a hospital-centric system, it became apparent that standardised clinic care and a reactive mode of care delivery of referrals are insufficient to treat mental illness and to promote the mental well-being of our youth.

Let us take an analogy from the evolution in the banking sector. In the past, consumer banking emphasised on bank branches in selected locality and human-teller interface. Now it has transformed to serving customers via a dense network of Automated Teller Machines (ATMs) and online banking through the Internet. Information and service were pushed right into the homes of the consumer or the mobile device of the consumer who is on the move. The consumer, in turn, interacts and provides inputs to the bank at the point of need for the service and receives service instantaneously. Banking service delivery has revolutionised over the past decades and successfully reached out to huge numbers of consumer banking users, serving them with more targeted service and personalised attention. The complexity of care and treatment of the mental well-being of a child or an adolescent parallels that of delivering banking service to the consumer — it requires targeted service and personalised attention.

We remain cognisant that fully automated service is not appropriate, at least not in the foreseeable future — given the general agreement that human clinical judgment remained an essential component of care and treatment. Our population-based model of care envisions that the mental well-being of a child and adolescent is not confined to the geographical premises of clinics and hospitals (except for tertiary care) but is characterised by "Service-at-the-doorstep" (much like the ATM is to the bank user) i.e. providing accessibility and convenience at the natural setting of the child/adolescent, and at a timing that optimises preventive care and early intervention for the individual.

This community-centric personalised care model comprises five essential operating criteria:

Effectiveness: Good enough care

Mental and emotional health refers to the presence of positive characteristics in the way one thinks, feels and acts as one copes with his or her life. It also helps determine how one handles stress, relates to others and makes choices (Institute of Mental Health [IMH], 2012). Mental healthcare that is "good enough" would be reflected through addressing the multi-faceted needs of the population to maintain good mental health, identifying mental health disorders early, and establishing a comprehensive intervention programme in primary, secondary and tertiary healthcare settings (Asia Australia Mental Health, 2011). While the intervention programme should serve the population as a whole, it would not be imposing "standardised" treatment on individuals. Rather, it should involve firstly, identification — based on accurate assessment — of the multiple, systemic factors which contribute to the mental health issues of the individual and secondly, leveraging on a network of community resources, each with different specialty, to effect a personalised management and treatment programme for the individual.

Accessibility: a pull vs. push system

The typical tertiary mental healthcare setting is a *Pull* system. It receives referral and provides treatment as the expert, with a black-box effect, as its services are often not easily understood. The psychiatric institution, as a provider of services, is traditionally shunned by the population, till a point when problems become complex and severely impairing the individuals. Often, by this stage, some damages are irreversible, and this tends to perpetuate the stigma against approaching the institution for help earlier.

The mental healthcare service for children and adolescents should be a *Push* system so as to enable early preventive and intervention efforts for this group of young population. The *Push* model raises the accessibility of mental healthcare services by means of a mobile multidisciplinary team, which is connected to schools, family doctors and social service agencies within the community. The team would collaborate closely with these parties to deliver an integrated management and treatment programme for the child or adolescent.

Timeliness: Just in time care

In Singapore, the education system, the primary healthcare system and the social service system are the three main first-line contact for children and adolescents. It is intuitive to tap on the school personnel (e.g. counsellors, teachers) and social service providers to conduct early screening and triage, so as to identify the risks and early signs of mental health distress. This timeliness in identification would initiate early intervention to prevent aggravation and more complex and costly treatment, and ideally, enable preventive interventions to enhance the coping capacity, and in turn, the mental well-being of the children and adolescents.

Affordability: Value for money care

Through linking the family and the child or adolescent to resources that already exist in their natural environment, care and treatment could take place within the community, rather than in the tertiary setting. There is no need to tax the tertiary care system, which is costly.

Safety: Do-no-harm care

Pushing mental healthcare services to the community, instead of centralising such services at the tertiary setting, is by no means compromising the quality of service or the safety of the population. The principles of beneficence and non-maleficence must be observed.

REACH — A step towards community-centric model of care

REACH, a mobile mental health team that operates in collaboration with community agencies including schools, general practitioners, and voluntary welfare organisations was conceptualised in alignment with the population-based model. In 2007, REACH was set up as one of the four pillars of the National Mental Health Blueprint, with a target population of children and adolescents below 19 years old.

The objectives of REACH include:

i) Improve the mental health of children in the community, with a focus on schools
ii) Provide early intervention through the support and training of school counsellors, social service agencies and voluntary welfare organisations in managing at-risk children
iii) Develop a mental health network in the community to support children at risk, involving voluntary welfare organisations, general practitioners and community pediatricians and schools

The mobility of REACH enables accessibility to mental health assessment and intervention, where students at risk of mental health illnesses are identified at the point of need i.e. in schools, student care service and at home. Youths-at-risk who may not be in school are identified through their engagements with restorative programmes and other assistance provided by community agencies. Collaborative interventions between REACH and help workers at these agencies would enable the youths to receive mental health assessment and treatment on-site. Combining the help worker's knowledge of the child or adolescent, and the professional know-how of the REACH team, the child or adolescent would receive more targeted service and personalised care, thus resulting in a better outcome.

Operationalising the community-centric model of care

The community-centric model of care is operationalised through close collaboration among multiple parties — from school counsellors, educators, youth workers, social service agency case workers, to primary healthcare professionals, mental health workers, child protection officers, police officers and youth rehabilitation workers. The services and the contribution of the professionals are multi-faceted and interdependent and involve different points of entry and at varied timings. Their collaboration could be direct, where one agency or party works in tandem with another, such as the case of the school counsellor helping a student referred by his teacher, or indirect, such as a social worker at a Voluntary Welfare Organisation (VWO) running youth programmes for school-going children of low-income parents. In order that this model of care delivery is effective, it is imperative that such collaboration is *multi-sectoral, multi-agency and multidisciplinary*.

Collaboration across sectors: The whole-of-government approach

Mental health and mental well-being is not just a Health Ministry issue. As primary school education is mandatory, schools form the most appropriate avenue for preventive and intervention efforts. Children and adolescents who are educated in schools that support their special needs, as well as those who are out-of-school, are also target beneficiaries of the mental health services. The management of mental health for children and adolescents involve various touch-points within the education system, the social service system, the corrective system, etc. It is necessary to engage these children who are at risk of behavioural and emotional disturbance (including violence), and their families, before the emerging problems become severe. It is therefore imperative that key agencies in the government, namely Ministry of Health (MOH), Ministry of Education (MOE), then-Ministry of Community Development, Youth and Sports (MCYS)/ National Council of Social Service (NCSS), Juvenile/Family Court and the Singapore Police Force, collaborate to achieve the common goal of improving the mental well-being of our children and adolescents.

Collaboration across agencies: A multi-agency network

The REACH teams

To serve the young population in Singapore, three hospitals- the Institute of Mental Health (IMH), the National University Hospital (NUH), and the KK Women's and Children's Hospital (KKH) are identified to host the REACH mobile teams which provide island-wide services. In total, the REACH teams will be servicing more than 350 schools.

The Partners of REACH

The REACH team seeks to partner with hundreds of VWOs that serve children and adolescents in different geographical zones, and at a national level. Some of these VWOs include the Singapore Children's Society (Yishun FSC), Persatuan Persuratan Pemuda Pemudi Melayu (4PM), Beyond Social Services, Students Care Service (Hougang and Clementi), MCYC Community Services Society and Fei Yue FSC (Yew Tee, Bukit Batok and Choa Chu Kang). Another segment of the community mental health network comprises the GPs who support primary healthcare at different residential districts.

Integrating effect of REACH

REACH conducts systematic assessment that integrates information from multiple agencies that were involved at different times of the child's development; and it also activates multiple agencies in the care and management of the child and adolescent.

Examples

- Management and interventions for an adolescent with mood symptoms, at-risk behaviours and challenging familial and parenting issues could involve KKH/NUH, IMH, VWO, neighbourhood police post, school, then-MCYS and children's home.
- Treatment and care for a child with anxiety symptoms and problematic behaviours, and parental history of mental illnesses could involve KKH, NUH, IMH, VWO, school and then-MCYS.

Collaboration across disciplines: A multidisciplinary team

The REACH team adopts a bio-psychosocial and developmental model of assessment and intervention to address the multi-faceted issues of a child or adolescent. This would require various domains of community mental health expertise. By locating the various disciplines together to conduct assessment and develop care plan, the pitfalls of assessment blind spots or intervention silos could be avoided and evidence-based practice could be strengthened through sharing among the professionals. The clinical arm of the REACH team comprises psychologist, medical social worker (MSW), occupational therapist (OT), community psychiatric nurse and medical doctor.

Supporting the clinical expertise, executive and administrative assistant are instrumental in the operations of REACH services, including financing, and measurement of progress and outcomes, etc. The operations personnel and the clinical personnel of the REACH team are led by a programme director.

Refer to Appendix A for a description of the scope and focus of each role in the REACH team.

Case example: Marcus

Marcus is a 7 year-old Chinese boy attending primary 1 in school when he was referred to REACH for highly active and disruptive behaviour in school as well as absenteeism. Marcus' mother was his only caregiver. The REACH team conducted an assessment in their home. The team's mobility enabled observation and interaction with Marcus and his mother in their natural environment. The REACH team of assessors, comprising a medical officer and a medical social worker, gathered that Marcus was at-risk of Conduct Disorder associated with limitations in care-giving and parenting, and with triggers from emotional distress experienced by his mother. They were informed that this family was previously helped by the then-MCYS Child Protection Service. The REACH team convened a case conference in the school to explain the holistic assessment and coordinated a treatment plan which placed Marcus' behavioural issues in the context of his mother's mental health. The conference involved the school management and teaching staff, the school counsellors, then-MCYS Officers, social workers at a VWO from which Marcus and his mother had obtained help from, and a multidisciplinary team from REACH comprising a medical officer, a medical social worker and a psychologist. The effective coordination in planning care for Marcus' mental health and continued development demonstrated a multi-agency and multi-sectoral approach in REACH operation.

The REACH Model

The REACH model, encompassing different levels of collaboration based on five operating criteria of quality care, and a support mechanism involving regional health systems, is illustrated in Figure 1.

Community-centric personalised services

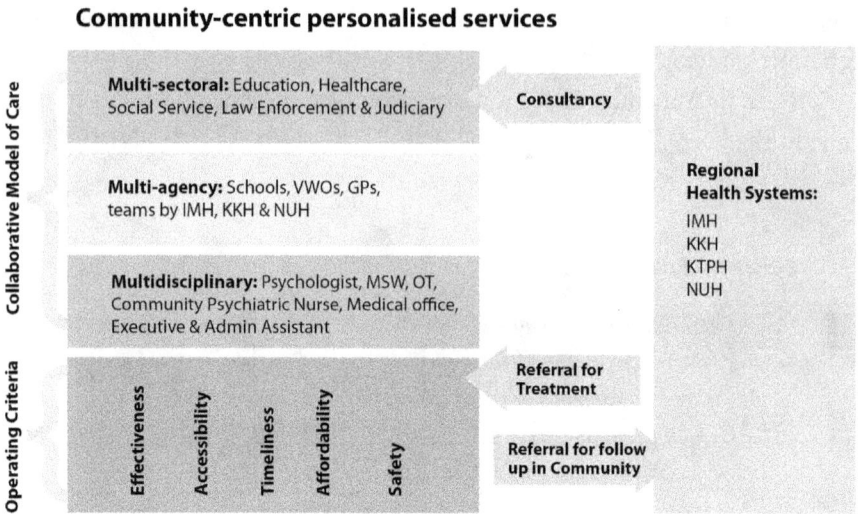

Figure 1. The REACH model for children and adolescents in Singapore

Core service

The core service of REACH is a helpline supported by a mobile team of multidisciplinary mental health professionals. The helpline aims to serve specific communities of professionals who come into contact with children and adolescents in their natural environments, namely school counsellors, service providers at voluntary welfare organisations, and family physicians. Referrals are made through this helpline, for assessment of mental health disorders as well as initiation of intervention by REACH. REACH operates a triage system for the referrals received to enable right-siting of care and early intervention.

Starting with Attention Deficit Hyperactivity Disorder (ADHD)

The project aims to increase the accessibility of support and intervention for students with emotional and behavioural difficulties, starting with ADHD. Children with ADHD belong to the largest category of mental health disorders that has been identified by WHO. It also represents the top diagnosis of conditions seen at the IMH's Child Guidance Clinic (CGC).

Children with this diagnosis typically require follow-up for an average of three to six years. REACH started out by collaborating with schools, GP and CGC for the management of children with ADHD. Involvement of GPs for treatment of this group of children is the first step in right-siting of care.

A phased-approach

A phased-approach was adopted in the processes and operation of REACH. In 2007, the first multidisciplinary team was set up by the Department of Child and Adolescent Psychiatry of IMH and MOE, as a prototype programme in a school cluster which consisted of 12 schools (including primary and secondary schools). Named the "GP — School Network Project", it aimed to train and support school counsellors in the early identification and support of children with behavioural and emotional difficulties. REACH was introduced under the collaborative effort between the IMH — CGC, and the Schools Division and then-Education Programmes Division of the MOE.

The first REACH team was formed to support 90 schools in the North zone. This team is located at the IMH which was close to schools in the northern part of Singapore in order to provide easy access and quick response. The second team was formed in 2009 to support schools in the south zone. The team is located in the southern part of Singapore and is also near the IMH's CGC at the Health Promotion Board. This enables REACH staff to manage referred REACH patients collaboratively with the clinical team at the CGC. The third REACH team opened in the east zone of Singapore in October 2010. The final team, situated in the west zone, was launched in March 2011.

The staggered effect of implementing REACH, as illustrated in Figure 2, allowed later teams to tap on the experience of earlier teams. The processes were refined iteratively as the MOE and IMH advanced through the zonal implementation for mainstream schools. Training programmes and materials for school counsellors were developed and enhanced throughout the five-year period as schools in more zones adopted the REACH services.

Year	Implementation with			
	GP	Mainstream schools	VWOs	SPED schools
2007		1 Cluster in North-zone	-	-
2008		North-zone	-	-
2009	On-going	South-zone	-	-
2010		East-zone	4 pilot agencies	-
2011		West-zone		4 pilot schools

Figure 2. Implementation of REACH teams to support schools in sequence of geographical regions

Furthermore, REACH helpline was offered to VWOs in 2010 and 2011, and by that time, the processes and operations of REACH were refined and became more comprehensive. While REACH was implemented in phases, recruitment and training of GP partners took place as an ongoing effort.

The funding of REACH

The Singapore healthcare financing system is anchored on the twin philosophies of individual responsibility and affordable healthcare for all. During the initial five-year roll-out of REACH starting from 2007, it receives full funding from the Ministry of Health. This is necessary to achieve increased awareness and outreach of mental health and to build capabilities in community resources. Following the first five years, funding will be allocated to hospitals responsible for the REACH teams based on a cost-recovery framework. To achieve cost recovery, REACH will offer services on a charging model, with fees kept at affordable rates. Financial assistance schemes will be made available to those who need them, so that cost will not be a key deterrent for the public to come forward and seek help. Nevertheless, mental health assessment conducted on the first visit by the REACH teams will still be kept free of charge to encourage parents to seek mental health help for their children.

Towards a vision of community-centric personalised services

The REACH model seeks to meet its operating criteria in accessibility, effectiveness and timeliness through a collaborative model of mental healthcare that delivers the appropriate level of treatment and preventive interventions in a personalised and timely manner for children and adolescents in Singapore. REACH achieves these key qualities by means of a helpline that is readily accessible to various parties who are in first-line contact with children and adolescents, an effective triage system, and a multidisciplinary team of mental health professionals that is highly mobile and in close coordination with a wide and responsive network of community partners.

By supporting early identification and preventive care for at-risk children and adolescents that is community-based, REACH could bring about greater coordination and utilisation of community resources and raise the level of mental healthcare for this population. In place of unnecessary and costly hospital-based treatment, the operation of REACH as a community-based service aims to provide appropriate and quality care that is affordable and founded on principles of "do-good" and "do-no-harm", via a referral mechanism with tertiary-level psychiatry consultancy.

To achieve the vision of REACH, a crucial effort would be the development of efficient and effective processes that uphold the operating criteria and put the collaborative model of care into practice. These outreach clinical services would in turn be facilitated by processes which raise the mental health competency of helping professionals in the community, and processes that facilitate the collaboration and networking of the REACH partners in the community, as illustrated in the subsequent chapters.

Our Multidisciplinary REACH Teams

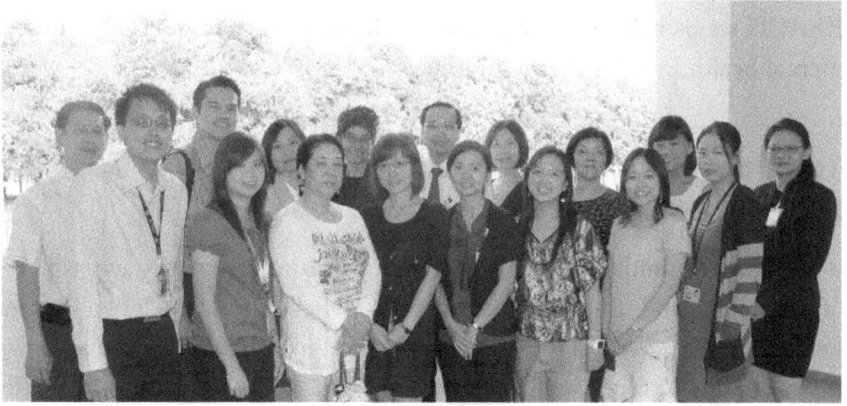

REACH North team (2011)

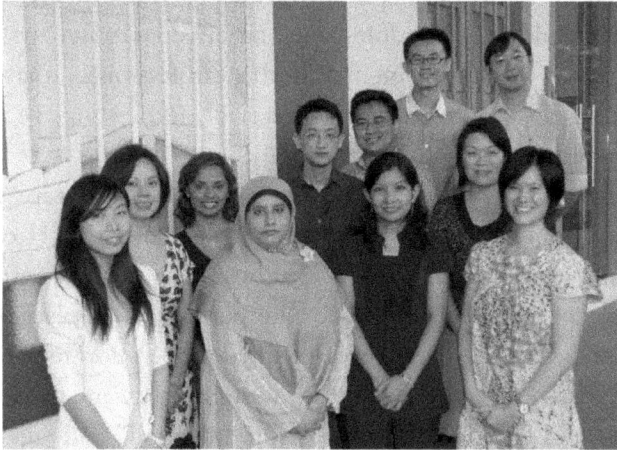

REACH South team (2011)

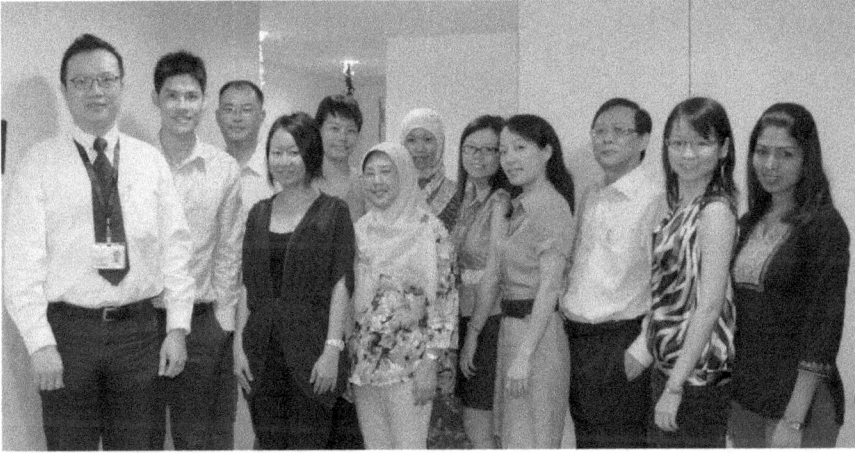

REACH East team (2011)

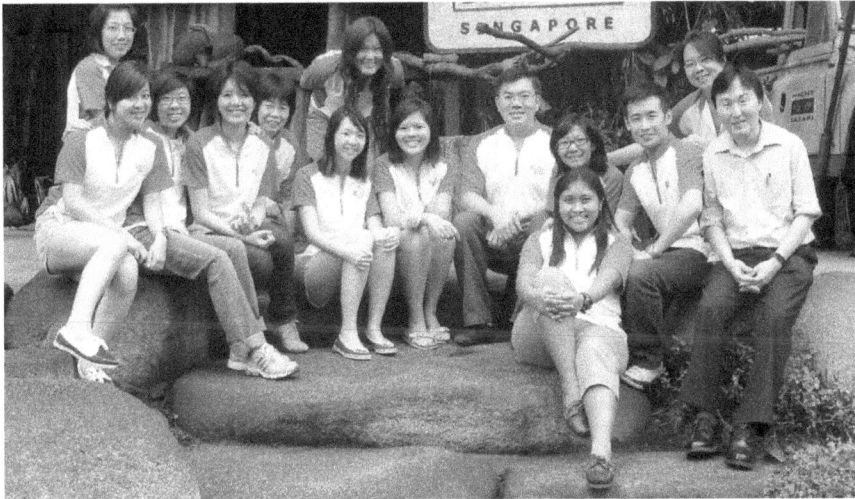

REACH West team (2011)

Chapter 2

Mental Health OutREACH: Processes and Services

Cheryl Lee

To reach out to children and adolescents who require mental health care in the community, REACH services need to be effective in two key areas: Firstly, facilitating referrals to REACH and providing appropriate and timely advice, and secondly, providing appropriate mental health training for helping professionals with whom children and adolescents have first-line contact, as well as the networking of community resources (Fung, Chua & Wong, 2011).

It needs to be highlighted that the effectiveness of *training and networking* has a relevant and direct impact on the effectiveness of REACH *referral and advice*. By enhancing the knowledge and skills of helping professionals (including school counsellors in mainstream schools, social workers and counsellors in VWOs, and psychologists in special education schools) in issues of mental health concerning children and adolescents, the helping professionals achieve a higher accuracy in identifying children and adolescents that require specialised mental health treatment. This reduces unnecessary referrals at the REACH helpline and allows REACH resources to be channelled to appropriate cases requiring specialised mental health care. At the same time, the less severe problems could be addressed earlier by appropriate resources in the community (Ooi *et al.*, 2012).

The relevance of enhancing networking among community resources, on the other hand, is that it enables quicker and closer collaboration among the community agencies due to the relationships established via partnerships with REACH. It can lead to greater corroborative knowledge about the child or adolescent who needs help, which is crucial for more effective assessment and generation of more relevant options and plans to assist the child and his or her family (Fung & Lim-Asworth, 2012).

Referral & advice

Referral

REACH provides its services to schools, VWOs and GPs via a helpline. The helpline is accessible to the school counsellor or the VWO staff via facsimile, electronic mail or phone. REACH personnel are scheduled daily to monitor the REACH helpline and address the enquiries and referral requests received. Figure 1 summarises the workflow by which mainstream schools refer children and adolescents who have emotional and behavioural issues and require mental health assessment by REACH. SPED schools and VWOs identify children and adolescents that require mental health assessments with different internal processes, but adopt a similar workflow to refer to REACH. Figure 2 illustrates the overall workflow that SPED schools and VWOs adopt.

As the referral processes adopted by SPED schools and VWOs are similar to that used by mainstream schools, references made to schools and school counsellors would also be taken to include SPED schools/VWOs and their respective staff.

A set of principles of care and assessment underlies the processes involved from the time the school identifies a potential student for referral to the time the student receives the necessary support. These are illustrated as follows:

The school support team

Secondary Schools and Junior Colleges are encouraged to form a School Support Team comprising the school counsellor, Allied Educator trained in Learning and Behavioural Support (AED [LBS]), school management personnel (e.g., vice principals and heads of departments), teachers trained in Special Needs (TSNs) and other key personnel identified by the school

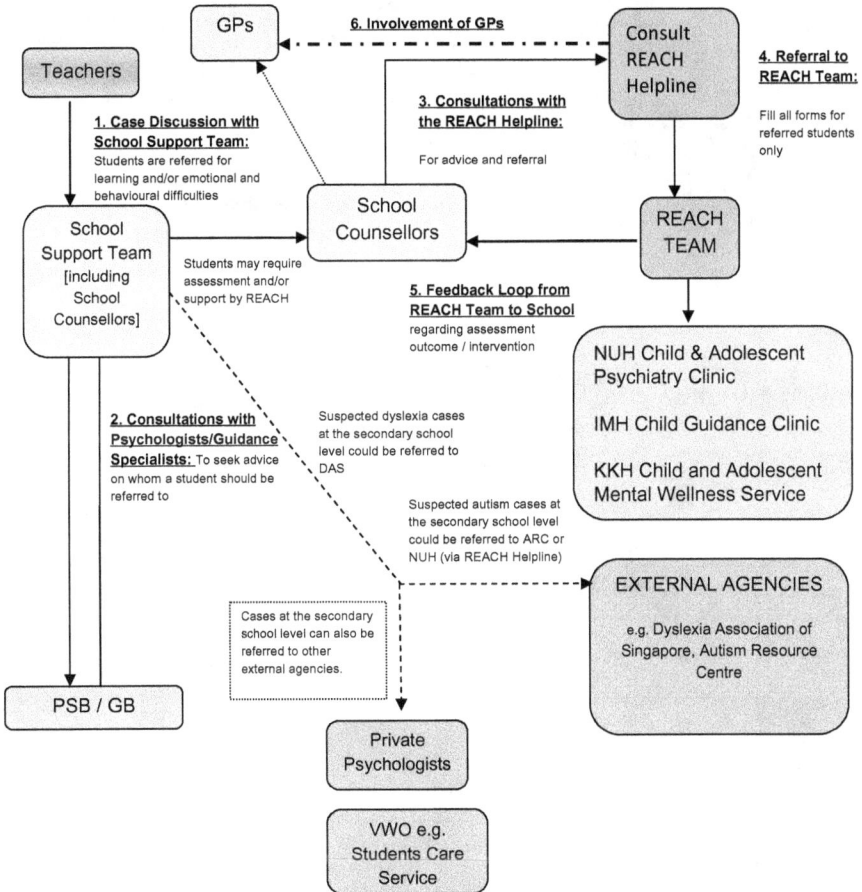

Figure 1. Referral Workflow for Children in Mainstream Schools Identified with Mental Health Issues

principal. This team serves the four-fold purpose of providing consultation to teachers who seek support for students in their classes, making referrals to REACH, monitoring the outcome of referrals and subsequently providing feedback to teachers and REACH on progress of cases. In the case of primary schools, a pre-existing Case Management Teams would serve the function of the School Support Team to collaborate with REACH. The school is responsible for planning and implementing school-wide support programmes and providing advice to staff and parents, usually through the Allied Educators.

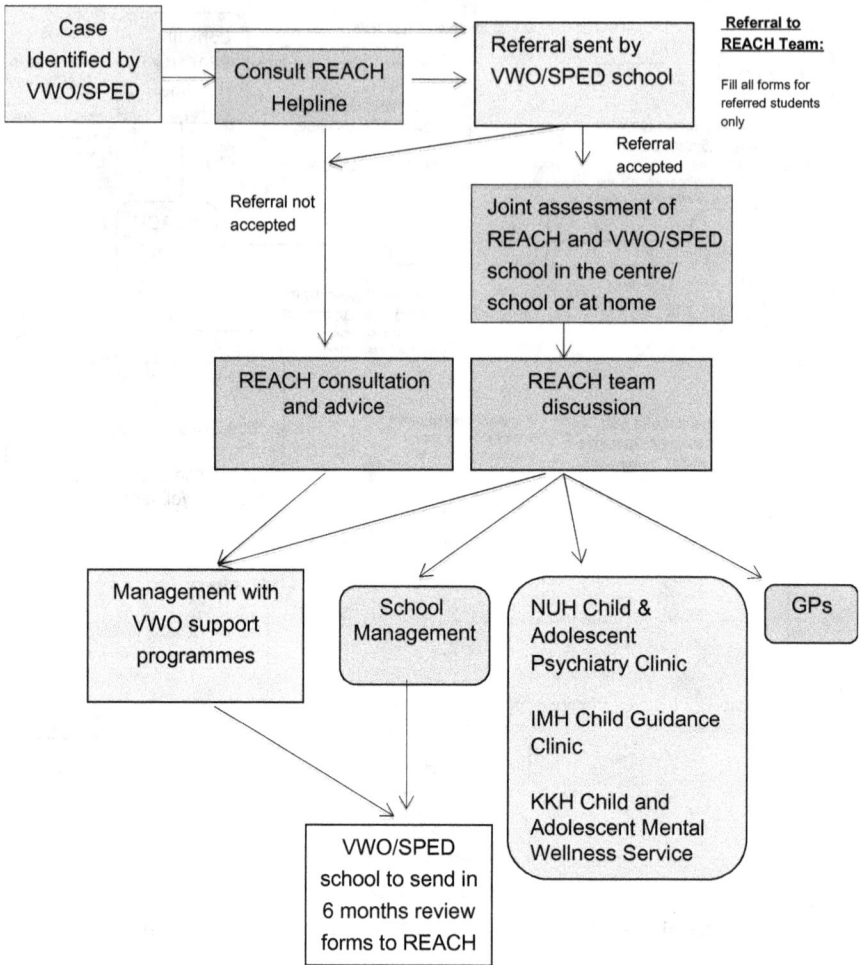

Figure 2. Referral Workflow for Children in the community and SPED suspected of mental health issues

Identification & initiation of referral

Teachers highlight potential cases to the School Support Team for discussion and potential referral to REACH. Identified students may have learning and/or emotional and behavioural difficulties. At this point, suggestions for behavioural intervention and support may be offered by the School Support Team.

Students with mild to moderate emotional and behavioural problems are helped by the school counsellors. The psychologists from Psychological Services Branch are consulted in the event of suspected learning difficulties (e.g., dyslexia) and they provide learning assessments for students in primary school. Where a mental health issue is suspected (e.g., suspected ADHD with learning difficulties, depression, eating disorders), the School Support Team makes the decision to refer the student to REACH.

The school counsellor consults the REACH Helpline to determine the suitability of the case for referral. The school counsellor then completes a triage form detailing the presenting problem and background of the student. In some cases, the referral may be triaged over the phone by REACH personnel, with the school counsellor providing the required information.

The information gathered upon triage includes a detailed history of the presenting problem (i.e., onset, frequency, duration and severity of the problem), family background and the school's main concern for the student. It is also important to establish whether the family is agreeable to the referral and whether there is an immediate risk of harm to the student (e.g., abuse or suicide risk). This enables the team to make adequate consideration of the case for acceptance.

Acceptance of referral

Cases are formally accepted by REACH after discussion at Case Management Rounds. For acceptance, cases generally need to constitute issues of a mental health nature and the student in question needs to be a registered student of the school. Cases that are not accepted (e.g., learning difficulties without other mental health issues) are channelled to the relevant organisations (e.g., Dyslexia Association of Singapore) for help. School personnel are provided with advice on where to proceed for help on the case.

For cases that are accepted, school counsellors proceed to obtain written parental consent and prepare the documents to process the referral. Required forms are submitted prior to the initial assessment conducted by REACH.

The forms, filled in by different parties, include the Clinical Global Impressions (CGI), the Strengths and Difficulties Questionnaire (SDQ) and the Euro-Quotient 5 Dimension (EQ-5D). These screening tools completed at baseline provide a gauge of the student's challenges and current state as reported by the school counsellor, parents and student. The teacher is also required to fill in the school report form which requires information on the student's behaviour in class and academic capabilities. These forms allow for comprehensive and standardised information gathering prior to the initial assessment. The team developed this process over time and has made many attempts to keep the paperwork to a minimum without sacrificing the objective of having this pre-assessment.

REACH Categorisation of Referrals

The timeliness of action depends on case severity and type. This is detailed in Table 1. Some cases (e.g., active self-harm behaviour) can be seen within a day of referral. Initial assessment must be done within a month of the referral.

Table 1. Categorising cases by severity determines the action taken for each case

Category	Action
Category 1: Presence of immediate risk to self or others (e.g., suicidal patient)	Assessed by REACH on the day itself if the student can be seen within office hours before deciding on need to transfer to Institute of Mental Health for admission. If the student can only be seen after office hours, the school and parents are advised to be seen at the Emergency Services at the Institute of Mental Health
Category 2: Disruptive behaviour affecting others. Serious problem with no immediate safety concerns or medical problems (e.g., student with high but no immediate risk of suicide)	Seen by REACH team within a week
Category 3: Non-disruptive behaviour confined to self. No immediate safety or medical problems	Seen by REACH team within a month
Category 4: Students not presenting with mental health issues	REACH team to recommend help at other agencies that are appropriate for the student's non mental health problems

Case example

Sean is an 8 year-old student referred to Amy, the school counsellor, by Sean's teacher. His parents were concerned about Sean's consistently poor grades. His form teachers described him as a fidgety boy who often walked around the classroom while lessons were going on. His attention span was short and he required constant prompting to redirect his attention. He did not get along with his peers and was quarrelsome and disruptive in class. Sean's parents also shared that he did not sit still for long at home and was often up and about. Amy also gathered some basic information on his family make-up, parents' age and occupation. There were no recent stressors in the family.

Amy discussed Sean's case with the School Support Team and they suggested some strategies to support Sean in the classroom. After trying them out for two weeks, Sean's form teacher reported minimal improvement. The School Support Team then agreed to refer the case to REACH.

With the information she had gathered, Amy called the REACH helpline to refer Sean to REACH for assessment. The REACH member on Helpline duty went through the REACH Triage Form with Amy and filled out the relevant sections. The REACH member then discussed the case with the REACH team, who agreed to see Sean and his parents for a mental health assessment at school. Internally, Sean's problem was seen as a category 3 problem as there was no serious risk of harm to self or others. In the meantime, Amy prepared the relevant forms for REACH assessment and faxed to the REACH office before the day of the REACH assessment.

On-site assessment

Where possible, assessment by REACH is carried out in the school setting together with the student, family and school counsellor. This allows for corroboration of information which is necessary for a more holistic assessment.

During the assessment, more information about the presenting issue is gathered from all parties. There is a systematic review of the student's sleep, appetite, compulsions and defiant behaviours. Details of the student's family history, past psychiatric history, and personal history are gathered at the assessment. Schooling, medical and social history are also explored during the interview. Parental expectations are a vital component of the interview. An examination of the student's mental state is carried out as part of the assessment.

The multidisciplinary nature of the REACH team is particularly helpful during the on-site assessments because personnel of each discipline can be called upon to provide assessments where appropriate (e.g., occupational therapist assessments and psychological assessments).

The REACH team routinely carries out home visits, classroom observations, discussions with VWOs and other external parties as part of initial assessment. This is to facilitate a holistic assessment of the case and varies according to the nature of each case.

Feedback loop & case management

Cases are systematically formulated based on the Diagnostic and Statistical Manual of Mental Disorders, fourth edition, text revision (DSM-IV-TR) and the 7Ps (i.e., Presenting problems, Predisposing factors, Precipitating factors, Perpetuating factors, Protective factors, Plan and Prognosis). Diagnoses and treatment plans are consulted with and endorsed by consultant psychiatrists to ensure a high standard of care for those under the team's care.

Feedback on all initial assessment outcomes is provided by the REACH team. REACH arranges for case conferences involving all key stakeholders in a case through the school counsellors. The case conference discussion includes the confirmed diagnoses (if any) and treatment plan for possible follow-up action or monitoring. REACH places emphasis on holistic management of cases and strives to involve all key stakeholders in carrying out the treatment plan.

If specialised care is required, REACH makes a referral for the student to be seen by mental health professionals at NUH Child & Adolescent Psychiatry Clinic, KKH Child and Adolescent Mental Wellness Service or IMH Child Guidance Clinic. These services are chargeable. Further long-term follow-up management can be provided by the school, family or other external agencies. For example, REACH may recommend that a student be referred to a mentoring programme available at a Family Service Centre. REACH can also provide assistance in the form of co-therapy with the school counsellor. The management of each case is a collaborative effort that hinges on early assessment (provided by REACH) and timely intervention (provided by key stakeholders and relevant external agencies).

Case example (*Continued*)

Two weeks following the acceptance of the referral, Sean, his parents and Amy met with the REACH team in school for an on-site assessment. A thorough history was obtained, which suggested that Sean's inattention and hyperactivity were evident since nursery school. Sean was also described as being fidgety, restless, and impatient at home and in other social settings. There was no family history of mental illness and the family was intact and supportive. Based on the thorough assessment conducted, Sean's condition fulfilled the criteria for Attention Deficit Hyperactivity Disorder (Combined type).

Sean's case was presented to the REACH team and consultant psychiatrist and the impression was that Sean's presenting difficulties were consistent with a diagnosis of ADHD. Sean's parents had sent him for cognitive testing prior to the referral, hoping to account for his poor grades. The results of the test suggested average cognitive functioning, indicating that his poor results were not likely to be due to his cognitive ability. Sean was referred to a psychiatrist to be treated for ADHD. In addition, REACH carried out psycho-education and shared some behavioural management strategies with Sean's teachers and parents. REACH continued to monitor Sean's progress for a period of six months, during which he showed improvement in most subjects and was observed to share better relationships with his peers and teachers.

Follow-up care

Regular updates between the school and REACH team ensure that the treatment plans are carried out smoothly and progress is monitored. After six months, teachers, school counsellors and the student complete the SDQ, CGI and EQ-5D again respectively. These forms are also completed for cases that were referred to GPs or hospital. The forms provide a measurable gauge of the child's progress and allow the REACH team to determine if further treatment or a revision of the treatment plan is needed.

Helpline enquiries & advice

School counsellors are encouraged to consult the REACH helpline for information or advice even if they have not made a formal referral for the student. In cases where school counsellors are unable to obtain parental consent or if timely advice is needed prior to the assessment, the REACH helpline provides a good platform to brainstorm ideas and to provide suggestions on how to manage a particular student (with no identifying information reported). Queries raised by school counsellors can also be tabled for team discussion and the outcomes communicated to the school. GPs and VWOs also have access to the helpline which provides support for case discussion and general advice.

Training and networking

Beyond the formal referral process, REACH supports schools by giving talks and organising training for school counsellors. REACH teams also conduct regular visits to schools and provide a platform for networking and collaboration between mental health agencies, schools and other community agencies.

School visits

Even though the school counsellor is usually the main point of contact between REACH and the school, it is vital for the School Support Team and school leaders to be aware of REACH and its services. Regular visits are made to each school to introduce the REACH team and processes, and to address any general queries that school personnel may have. Such visits help establish a collaborative relationship between REACH and the school, thus easing the referral process. The visits also allow REACH team to understand the mental health needs of the individual schools and to tailor their support based on the requirements of the school.

On-going training for school counsellors

By inviting expert speakers to conduct training sessions on specific topics (e.g., ADHD and its management) or engaging REACH personnel to provide workshops and seminars (e.g., Depression or managing children with anger issues), schools are ensured of an on-going capacity building process that allows school counsellors and REACH teams alike to familiarise themselves with information and development of mental health issues as they unfold in our school system. Training for school counsellors aim to equip them with a variety of skill sets as they continue to be at the front line of mental healthcare in schools. After the school counsellors are trained, they are also supported to train other school personnel so as to create a ripple effect of mental health knowledge in the community.

REACH networks

Apart from close links with mainstream schools, REACH has also established working links with GPs, VWOs and SPED Schools (Institute of Mental Health, 2011).

Interagency case conferences and discussions are often organised for cases involving multiple agencies. During these case conferences, a common platform is established, allowing all parties to synergise their efforts through mutual discussion and sharing of information. This also reduces duplication of services provided.

REACH networks also allow referrals to be made by REACH to GPs and VWOs where appropriate. Students are able to approach GPs who have been identified in the GP network. GPs may see stable cases that require regular follow-ups such as ADHD, mood or anxiety disorders. The process for referring students to GPs is described in Chapter 5 — Partnership with GPs.

VWOs collaborating with REACH are also given access to the REACH helpline and can refer cases to REACH for early assessment and intervention. Conversely, REACH consults VWOs on cases that may be more suitable to be handled by VWO services. For example, VWOs may be better equipped to handle students that have dropped out of mainstream education (i.e. Out of School Youths). Further details on the partnership with VWOs are described in Chapter 4 — Partnership with VWOs.

Resources and relevant materials are commonly shared among VWOs, GPs and REACH. These parties are invited to trainings organised by REACH. Information sharing helps to promote growth and a common interest among these key organisations.

In summary, this chapter highlights the key processes involved in the referral process. It also elucidates the various platforms in place that encourage continuous capacity building and networking between REACH and VWOs, GPs and schools.

Supporting Schools: Strengthening the First Line of Defence for Students with Mental Health Difficulties

Wong Hui Yi and July Lies

Under the auspices of the National Mental Health Blueprint and a partnership between the MOH and the MOE, the REACH programme was launched in a cluster of 12 mainstream schools in 2007. Five years on, the REACH programme is now available in more than 350 schools in Singapore. This chapter explores the need for mental health initiatives to include schools as a major stakeholder, as well as reports on the progress of the REACH programme in mainstream and SPED schools, respectively.

A need for a partnership between the mental health and education systems

In Singapore, most children undergo at least ten years of general education, of which six years of primary school education is compulsory except for certain categories such as children with special needs, for whom other educational arrangements may be considered (MOE, 2012a). Thus, schools are an opportune site for the prevention, detection, and intervention for mental health problems in school-aged children and adolescents. Mental health and learning are also closely intertwined and students who have good mental health are more likely to achieve their academic potential, have fewer emotional and behavioural problems, have more meaningful relationships with others, and in general succeed later on in life and become responsible and constructive citizens. In contrast, risk factors associated with the school setting such as difficulties in coping with the academic curriculum and poor school attendance are commonly implicated in the development and maintenance of emotional and behavioural problems for children and adolescents (WHO, 2005). In addition to poor academic performance, students with poor mental health tend to have difficulties relating to others, have a negative sense of self, and poorer coping skills (Hendren, Weisen, & Orley, 1994). Thus, mental health services and schools have to work closely to provide a concerted response to optimise students' mental health and learning potential.

Before REACH was implemented in 2007, students' mental health needs were mainly served by hospital-based specialist clinics (e.g., Child Guidance Clinic [CGC] at IMH and the psychiatry departments in general hospitals). Schools would refer students with perceived mental health needs directly to these clinics, as did polyclinics, GPs and community agencies, and this resulted in a bottleneck situation at these clinics. Waiting times were long and cases were seen on a first-come-first-served basis with no triaging of the level of need for assessment and intervention. Some parents did not give consent for clinic staff to work with schools and even for those who did, actual communication and collaboration tended to be ad-hoc and inconsistent. There was stigma associated with mental health and some parents and students were reluctant to come to the clinics for assessment or interventions. As such, there was an increasing need for a closer partnership between mental health services and schools. This need also coincided with a broader paradigm shift from institution-based to community-based mental healthcare, the latter of which was associated with greater access and acceptability of mental healthcare services by the general population (WHO, 2003). The following two sections report on the implementation of the REACH model in mainstream and SPED schools, respectively.

REACH in Mainstream Schools

The landscape of mainstream schools in Singapore

Mainstream schooling in Singapore is served by 175 primary schools, 150 secondary schools, 13 mixed level (combined primary and secondary) schools, and 13 junior colleges (MOE, 2012b). The schools are divided into four regional zones (North, South, East and West) in combinations of primary, secondary and junior colleges. Each Zone has seven clusters of such school combinations of about ten to 15 schools. In each school, there is a school support team that works closely with teachers to support students with special educational needs and those with behavioural, social, and emotional issues. The school support team typically consists of school counsellors, allied educators trained in learning and behavioural support (AEDs [LBS]), teachers trained in special needs (TSNs) and school personnel in middle management (e.g., vice principals and heads of departments).

School counsellors are trained to support students with behavioural, social, and emotional issues and typically possess a Masters, postgraduate diploma, or diploma in counselling (MOE, 2012c). They are supported by supervisors from the Guidance Branch (GB), MOE and psychologists from the Psychological Services Branch (PSB), MOE. REACH was conceptualised to further support schools in the early detection and intervention for emerging mental health problems in students by offering advice and discussing referrals with school counsellors through the REACH Helpline, conducting clinical assessments and interventions for students, and training school counsellors on mental health topics.

Pilot phase of REACH in mainstream schools

In August 2007, the REACH prototype was piloted in twelve mainstream schools in one cluster of schools in the North zone (the then N1 cluster). This cluster of schools was chosen based on its proximity to IMH for easy access to the hospital's facilities and services. The main target population was initially students with ADHD and subsequently expanded to students with other mental health disorders between six and 18 years old who were

"It was an initial struggle to fill out the paperwork ... We were complaining about the paperwork, why do we need to fill up so many paperwork? ... Getting parents' consent was difficult too..."

Primary school counsellor, North zone

within the identified school cluster. A multidisciplinary mobile mental health team consisting of a psychiatrist, a trainee psychiatrist, nurses, psychologists, medical social workers, and an occupational therapist was created to work closely with school counsellors in this school cluster. The first REACH team led by Dr Daniel Fung was formed with experienced professionals from the wards and clinics in IMH. The team visited all the schools in the cluster to engage and build rapport with the school support teams. REACH services and processes were explained, the needs of schools were gathered, and feedback obtained was factored into improving our services and processes. For instance, instead of only accepting new referrals through the helpline, new referrals are now accepted through email and facsimile. The forms school counsellors were required to fill in for new referrals were reduced to capture essential information for assessment and evaluation. In addition to individual school visits, the REACH team joined the school counsellors at their cluster meetings with representatives from both PSB and GB in order to obtain feedback about REACH services and processes.

A REACH liaison person was appointed for each school to provide a single point of contact. The importance of a collaborative partnership between REACH and schools cannot be understated, as it is the platform for which early intervention, support, and training for mental health disorders is provided in the community. By end 2008, the REACH programme was extended to all schools in the North Zone. Over the next three years, the REACH programme was rolled out to schools in the South, East, and West Zones. Schools that were under the care of the respective REACH teams mirrored the zonal distribution of schools under MOE. The teams were also based in locations that would be most centralised for schools in their zones, as well as proximity to hospital-based Clinics for access to facilities and services. The following sections describe the various REACH services and some of our achievements and challenges thus far.

REACH Helpline: Advice and referrals of new cases

The impetus behind the REACH programme was to provide a more timely response to children with possible mental health issues. School counsellors are already supporting children with behavioural, emotional, and social issues and can refer those with learning issues to school personnel trained in special needs or consult MOE psychologists. However, they often need further support for children presenting with more complex mental health needs. The REACH Helpline is a dedicated service to school counsellors for advice and discussion of potential referrals to REACH, as well as progress of existing cases. New cases are triaged so as to ascertain the mental health issues and the level of urgency for REACH assessment and intervention. Figure 1 presents the number of calls to the REACH Helpline from 2007 to 2011 while Figure 2 shows the number of accepted school referrals to REACH from 2007 to 2011.

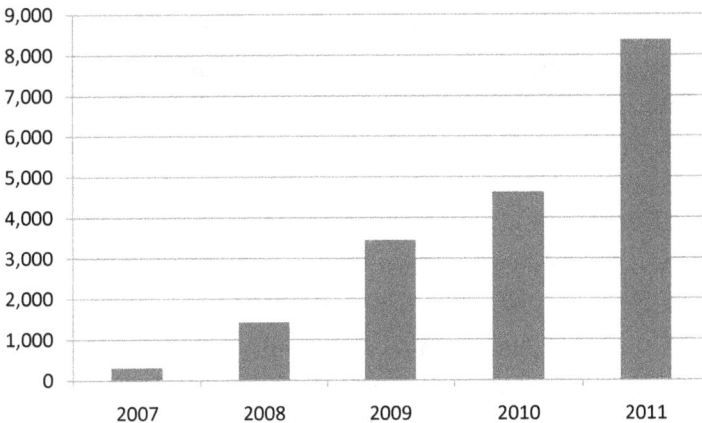

Figure 1.   Number of calls to REACH Helpline from 2007 to 2011

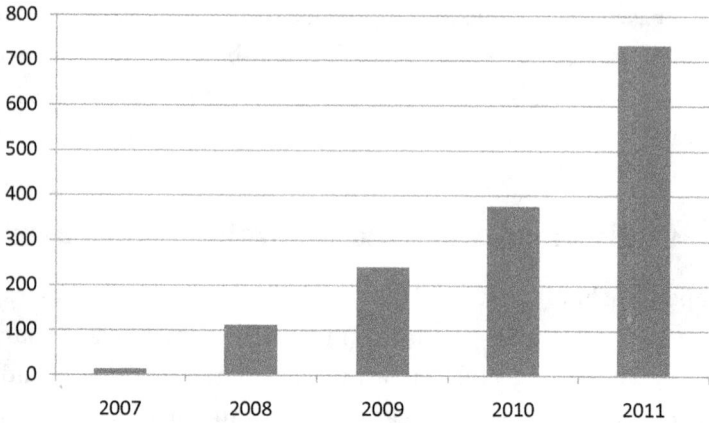

Figure 2. Number of accepted school referrals to REACH from 2007 to 2011

In tandem with the establishment of the respective REACH teams and the subsequent rollout of REACH services in the various zones, the number of calls to the REACH Helpline has risen steadily over the last five years (see Figure 1). The Helpline is a well-utilised REACH service and school counsellors have appreciated the immediacy and accessibility of advice and support via the Helpline. Similarly, the number of accepted school referrals to REACH has also increased over the last five years (see Figure 2). These numbers reflect the number of cases referred to and accepted by REACH for an assessment after the case is triaged at the Helpline stage. Many more cases are discussed and directed to the most appropriate site of care according to the needs of each case (e.g., school counsellor, MOE psychologist, and Family Service Centre). Over the last five years, 93% of all Category 2 cases and 99% of all Category 3 cases were seen by REACH within one week and one month, respectively. As compared to waiting times of at least three months for students to see the Clinic-based psychiatric team before REACH was formed, the waiting time to see the REACH team in the community is at most one month. This shorter waiting time is a testament to the responsiveness of the REACH team to every referred case, as well as the efficacy of a triage system in which the Helpline plays an integral role.

> "The designated REACH helpline makes it so much easier for seeking advice and making referrals from school. It is definitely a great help to talk to the REACH staff immediately without having to be put on hold or being referred to different persons."
>
> Secondary school counsellor, West Zone

REACH Assessments: Mental health assessments and beyond

On the day of assessment, a mental health assessment is conducted by one or two REACH members at the school or at the home, along with the school counsellor. The multi-disciplinary profile of every REACH team allows the selection of the appropriate personnel to conduct the assessment. Although all REACH personnel are trained mental health professionals, each REACH personnel is also cross-trained in the specific disciplines of psychiatry, nursing, psychology, social work, and occupational therapy. Discipline-specific skills and knowledge may be particularly useful and relevant for certain cases. For instance, if the case involves complicated family dynamics and suspected child abuse, the medical social worker may be assigned to the case, as his or her expertise in family therapy and child protection will come in handy. Where possible, REACH personnel who are proficient in particular languages are also assigned to certain cases based on the language preferences of the primary caregivers. The standard assessment entails interviewing parents and the student together, and then separately. The whole process takes about two hours, which includes interviewing the school

> "The collaboration between the school counsellor and the REACH team gives the school counsellor an opportunity to tap and gain expertise on the vast knowledge of mental (health) issues form the REACH team that consists of different mental health professionals."
>
> Primary school counsellor, South Zone.

53

counsellor and teachers (where available). A learning screen that covers basic literacy and numeracy skills is also conducted for primary school students who may have comorbid learning problems in addition to their mental health difficulties. Drawings and other checklists or rating scales of psychopathology (self/parent/teacher-report) may be used as well.

After the initial assessment, the case is formulated according to the "7Ps" (Presenting problems, Predisposing factors, Precipitating factors, Perpetuating factors, Protective factors, Plan, Prognosis) and presented to the team and consultant psychiatrist once a week. These case discussions tap on the various expertise of the multi-disciplinary team and a consensus is reached about diagnostic impressions and recommendations. At times, further assessments such as cognitive and academic assessments, classroom observations, home visits, and discussions with other medical or allied health professionals who have been involved in the case previously, may be required. After the assessment phase is completed, a feedback session is arranged with the school counsellor, parents, and may also involve students themselves to explain the student's mental health condition and the treatment plans and strategies.

Figure 3 shows a snapshot of the different types of mental health problems seen by the various REACH teams from March 2011 to March 2012 based on information gathered in the initial assessment. Behavioural problems include those relating to ADHD, Conduct Disorder, and Oppositional Defiant Disorder, and emotional problems include those relating to Mood and Anxiety Disorders. Developmental problems include those relating to Autism Spectrum Disorders and learning problems include those relating to learning disorders such as dyslexia. Other types of problems include school refusal, excessive computer usage, parent-child relational problems, and adjustment difficulties.

Figure 3 shows that more than half of cases seen by REACH pertained to either behavioural (33%) or emotional (20%) disturbances,

> *"The feedback sessions were good as the REACH team who came down for the feedback sessions made sure the parents understood what the situation was and how we can all work together to improve their child's life."*
>
> Primary school counsellor, East Zone

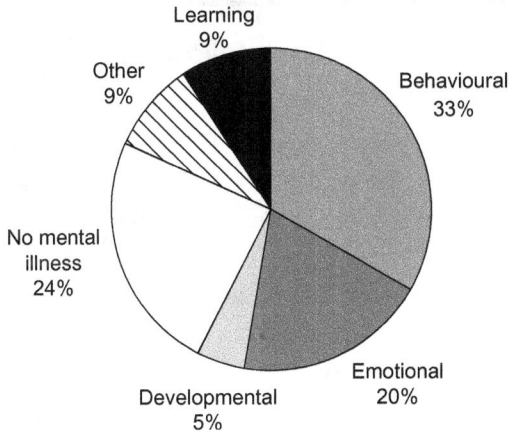

Figure 3. Types of mental health problems seen by REACH from 2011 to 2012

which is consistent with the main types of mental health problems exhibited by school-aged children and adolescents (WHO, 2005). A substantial proportion of students seen by REACH did not fulfil diagnostic criteria for a mental health disorder (24%). Some of these students may nevertheless be at risk of developing a mental health disorder at a later stage and would benefit from support and monitoring by school counsellors and/or REACH.

REACH-supported interventions and referrals to other services

Various options may be recommended following the initial REACH assessment and the principle is right siting of care depending on the level and type of care needed and according to evidence-based best practices.

For cases referred to the Clinic or to GPs, REACH helps to ease the transition by explaining to parents and students the Clinic process, as well as accompanying them for the first visit. Information obtained by REACH is made available to the doctors for their perusal with consent from parents and students. Apart from assessments and interventions, an important part of REACH work is in liaising with various partners such as schools,

---

Typical recommendations following the initial REACH assessment:

- Support school counsellors to conduct individual or group-based interventions for students such as teaching anger management and social skills, psychotherapy for depression or anxiety, activating school refusal protocols, or occupational therapy for handwriting or sensory issues.
- Support school counsellors to discuss behavioural management strategies with parents and teachers.
- Consult MOE psychologists regarding student's educational or learning needs.
- Refer students and their families to other service providers such as Family Service Centres for marital or family counselling or Youth Centres for outreach or after-school services and programs.
- Refer students to a GP partner for medication (See Chapter 5).
- Refer students to hospital-based mental health clinics for further assessment and interv entions, which may include medication, psychotherapy, family therapy, and/or occupational therapy.

MOE psychologists, GPs, VWOs, and other social agencies, as well as hospital-based Clinics. Over the last five years, a total of 1,437 case conferences were organised by the four REACH teams. Such liaison work facilitates the engagement of community partners and the development of a mental health network for children and adolescents in the community. All REACH cases are also reviewed six months after the date of the first REACH assessment so as to monitor the progress of each case. The efficacy of REACH-supported interventions depends in part on students', parents', and schools' abilities and consistency in carrying out the various recommendations. If there has been limited progress or improvements,

REACH reviews the treatment plans with school counsellors and relevant stakeholders. Depending on the needs of each case, these reviews tend to occur more frequently than the designated 6-month period and reflect the commitment of REACH in helping every student

"When it comes to interventions, sometimes they are effective and at other times, not. They are effective only when parents and students themselves apply what they have been taught. So far, the group sessions done in my school with REACH's help was the ALERT programme and the feedback from parents and students was good."

Primary school counsellor, South Zone

referred to us. The following case example of Gabriel illustrates how REACH helped him cope with his anxiety and how he eventually returned to school.

Case example: Gabriel

Gabriel is an 11 year-old Chinese boy who was referred for school refusal relating to his high level of anxiety about school. He was in Primary 5 at the point of referral. Based on information gathered in the assessment, the REACH team suspected that Gabriel was suffering from an anxiety disorder. The REACH team recommended for REACH and school counsellor be co-therapists and conduct school-based interventions, which included guided imagery and relaxation techniques and creating a calm and safe environment in the counsellor's room for Gabriel to go to when he was unable to cope with his anxiety. The REACH team also assisted in providing psychoeducation for Gabriel's parents to better understand his challenges, and parenting tips and strategies to better support Gabriel's return to school. A case conference was held with Gabriel's teachers so as to understand the challenges they face with supporting Gabriel, as well as help them better understand Gabriel's condition and how to support him in the classroom. With the support given at the individual, home, and school levels, Gabriel was eventually able to overcome his anxiety and return to school.

Benefits and challenges of school-based assessments and interventions

The flexibility and mobility of the REACH team is one of the greatest strengths of the REACH programme. Assessment and interventions can be done at schools or at home (when necessary) and at a time that is least disruptive to student's academic curriculum (where possible). For instance, the REACH team is able to help school refusal cases by conducting home visits in the morning before school starts to help students get to school on the day, with the support of their parents and the school counsellors. Additionally, the school is a naturalistic setting where most students feel comfortable and familiar, and are likely to feel less stigmatised seeking help for mental health issues as compared to a hospital setting. However, some may argue that some students and parents may prefer the anonymity and privacy of a hospital setting. Some students may feel uncomfortable being seen with the school counsellor and REACH personnel at school.

A major challenge faced by REACH in supporting school counsellors for interventions in school may lie in the student's motivation for change and adherence to therapy. In this regard, the ease and flexibility of which REACH-supported interventions are available at school could be a double-edged sword. While some students may be more open to seeking help because services are at their doorstep, others may not be ready to change and thus, may not engage in these services. For some students, their parents may not see the need for intervention or even an assessment in the first place since REACH referrals are typically initiated by school counsellors. Nevertheless, such a challenge is also an opportunity

> "REACH has provided students with a much needed access to mental health expertise in a setting which is child friendly and sensitive to community sentiments...Schools are now better equipped to assess, support, and manage students with mental health issues. REACH has allowed for more open channels of communication between family, school, and the mental health practitioners ..."
>
> Secondary school counsellor, South zone

to engage with students and parents who may otherwise not seek help from hospital-based clinics.

Mental health training for school counsellors

In the school system, school counsellors are the first port of call for teachers and parents who are concerned about students with emotional, behavioural, social and/or learning difficulties. MOE provides initial and ongoing training for all school counsellors and they are equipped to provide counselling to students and to provide case consultations to and training for school personnel and parents. REACH enhances counsellors' knowledge base and skill set in mental health by training them to recognise signs and symptoms of mental health disorders and to equip them with basic strategies and skills to deal with mild mental health issues. Training for school counsellors also reflects a 'train-the-trainer' approach where school counsellors can then create a ripple effect on mental health knowledge in the community by conducting training and providing consultations in their schools. Formal training is provided in a series of modular training that is organised by the REACH teams annually. These training sessions are publicised on a specialised website dedicated to school counsellors (See Chapter 6). Needs analyses were conducted with school counsellors in the respective zones to tailor training topics according to school counsellors' unique learning needs.

Example of training topics offered by REACH:

- Working with behavioural disorders in primary schools
- Working with behavioural disorders in secondary schools
- Working with school refusal cases
- Anger management for primary school students
- Medications & side effects
- Management of depression
- Triaging for mental health issues in schools
- ADHD for secondary school students
- Working with anxiety disorders in primary schools.

Over the last five years, a total of 997 school counsellors have attended 169 training sessions organised by the respective REACH teams. An overwhelming majority of school counsellors who have attended REACH training reported that the training has equipped them with the necessary skills to manage the students they see (97%) and that they are satisfied with the training provided (97%). However, increased knowledge on identifying and managing mental health conditions may not necessarily equate to increased confidence in school counsellors when they have to actually manage students with such conditions (Soo, Ong, Chen, & Ong, 2011). Much more has to be done to translate theoretical knowledge into practical skills and to build school counsellors' competencies and confidence in working with students with mental health issues.

In addition to training by REACH, overseas experts on child and adolescent mental health have also been invited to Singapore to provide training for school counsellors. Informal training is also provided via case discussions and working on cases together, as well as interagency case conferences conducted once a month

(At the interagency conferences), you get to see the support lent by different agencies, how to formulate hypotheses, challenges, how the case was presented. (It was) very useful.

Primary school counsellor, North zone

at CGC, HPB. Feedback from school counsellors with regard to factors contributing to their attendance at these training have indicated the importance of perceived relevance and applicability of topics to students they see in their schools. Personal interest is another oft-cited reason. Factors that have contributed to their non-attendance are mainly related to logistics and time constraints. Catering to different school counsellors with varying levels of experience and expertise is also a challenge. Newer school counsellors may prefer more generic training whereas more experienced ones may prefer more specialised training. Nevertheless, the overall feedback has pointed to the usefulness of REACH training for school counsellors in strengthening counsellors' abilities to detect signs of mental health disorders.

Improving children's mental health — Outcome data for mainstream schools

One of the main objectives of REACH is to improve children's mental health with a focus on schools by supporting school counsellors via the Helpline, conducting assessments and interventions, and by training them in mental health topics. In order to determine if children's mental health has improved after REACH involvement, data is collected on the following three measures on a six-month interval. All school counsellors are trained by REACH to either complete the relevant measure themselves or to administer the relevant measures to teachers or students.

Outcome measures

- The Strengths and Difficulties Questionnaire (SDQ) (Goodman, 1997) is a 25-item brief questionnaire that screens for behavioural and emotional problems in children and adolescents. The Total Difficulties score is computed from scores from four domains of emotional symptoms, conduct problems, hyperactivity, peer relationship problems. The SDQ is completed by a teacher who is familiar with the student.

- The Clinical Global Impression (CGI) (Guy, 1976) consists of two items – severity of illness and global improvement. Both items are rated on a 7-point scale with higher scores reflecting higher severity of illnesses and less improvement overall (i.e. getting worse), respectively. The CGI is completed by the school counsellor.

- The European Quality of Life — 5 dimensions (EQ-5D) (The EuroQol Group, 1990) consists of five items on mobility, self-care, usual activities, pain/discomfort, and anxiety/depression, and a visual analogue scale on perceived level of health state. The five items are rated on three levels — no problems, some problems, or extreme problems. The visual analogue scale is anchored by (0) — worst imaginable health state and (100) — best imaginable health state. The EQ-5D is completed by students aged 11 years and above.

Outcome data comparing students' overall level of emotional and behavioural problems at the time of the initial assessment by REACH and six months later have demonstrated a reduction in the level of these problems, according to teachers' and school counsellors' ratings, and self-report (where available). Koh, Sulaiman, Ooi, and Fung (2011) and Sulaiman, Ong, and Fung (2009) found significantly lower scores on all subscales of the SDQ and the CGI six months after students were referred to REACH. Preliminary analyses for an upcoming study by Koh and Boon (2012) have replicated these trends in a larger dataset involving about 700 students. Figure 4 shows the pre and post scores on the various SDQ subscales from this study.

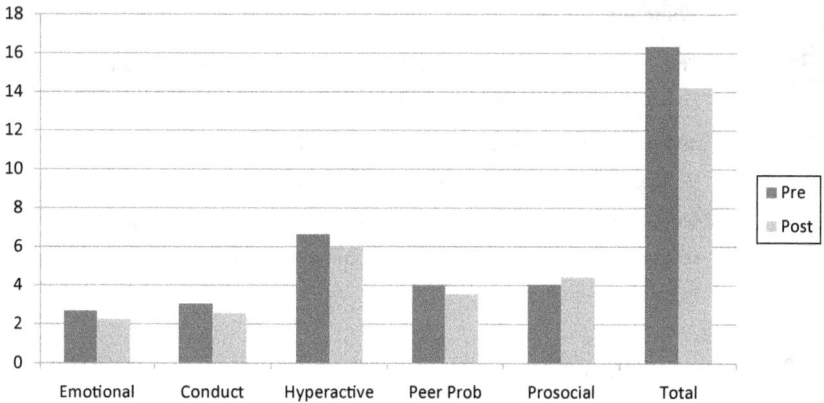

Figure 4. Pre and post teachers' ratings on SDQ subscales ($n = 690$)

Koh and Boon (2012) showed that on the SDQ, teachers reported significantly lower scores on the Emotional, Conduct, Hyperactive, Peer Problems, and Total Problems subscales, as well as higher scores on the Prosocial Behaviours subscale, six months after students were referred to REACH (see Figure 4). School counsellors also rated significantly lower scores on the CGI. Additionally, students themselves (those aged 11 years and older) reported better mobility, self-care, and ability to perform in usual activities, and lesser pain and discomfort and anxiety and depression on the EQ-5D. Students also rated themselves with significantly better overall health state on the visual analogue scale on the EQ-5D. In summary, analyses conducted to date have shown improvements in students' mental health six months after they were referred to REACH for an assessment. Students displayed fewer emotional, behavioural, and social problems, and were functioning better in different areas, according to different informants. Evidently, a closer look into the outcome data is required, which takes into consideration other factors such as diagnosis, type of intervention (e.g., REACH-supported intervention or referral to hospital-based mental health Clinics), and compliance and response to recommended intervention. Such investigations will shed light on the clinical effectiveness of the REACH programme and are currently underway.

Summary of REACH in mainstream schools

From providing advice and support to school counsellors over the Helpline, to conducting mental health assessments and interventions in schools, the majority (97%) of school counsellors have been satisfied with the support REACH has provided. Through REACH, students and parents are more likely to seek help for emerging mental health problems. By providing early intervention for these problems, the trajectory towards developing serious mental health problems may be prevented. Evidently, stigma is still a very real and relevant issue and despite REACH providing services in schools, some parents and students are still reluctant to engage REACH services. For some parents, the focus of their child is still overwhelmingly on academic performance. The task lies in greater awareness about mental health issues and the impact on children's learning and future development. Through REACH, schools are empowered to support students with mental health issues as specialised help is readily available. REACH processes from the point of contact at Helpline to assessment and interventions ensure that students with suspected mental health issues are seen and treated in a timely manner. Through REACH, community resources are tapped into and are part of a mental health network for children and adolescents. The safety net for the early detection and intervention for mental health problems is thus cast further and wider than the confines of the hospital-based Clinics.

"It's been an enriching experience working and collaborating with the REACH team for the betterment of the students referred. The constant updates and prompt feedback provides an environment of trust, and for the various stake-holders to respond appropriately. Their professional disposition and their caring attitude has been a source of encouragement to parents, students, and the school. The personal touch and support brings across the sincerity in wanting to help family and students with their challenges. Overall, a very positive engagement."

Secondary school counsellor, West zone

REACH in Special Education (SPED) Schools

Supporting schools

Education for school-going children and adolescents with special needs require a range of differentiated approaches in SPED schools. Depending on the type of special need and degree of impairment, some of these children and adolescents may be suited for mainstream schooling with additional support, while others may benefit from the specialised curriculum delivered in SPED schools.

The landscape of SPED schools in Singapore

SPED schools are operated by VWOs in partnership with MOE and NCSS. MOE and NCSS co-fund the resources and services to help these children and adolescents in SPED schools achieve a well-rounded education encompassing academic, independent living, social and pre-vocational skills. The broad aim of all SPED schools is to maximise the potential of each individual so as to promote their well-being and integration in the long run.

The special education curriculum not only equips the children and adolescents with the skills, knowledge and attributes required for community living, but also support their overall well-being through the various educational and therapy services. Besides classroom and community-based instructions by special education teachers, support is provided by a team of allied health professionals such as psychologists, speech therapists, occupational therapists, physiotherapists and social workers. Some of the commonly-occurring disabilities amongst the children and adolescents in Singapore include

Intellectual Disability[1]
Multiple disabilities[2]
Autism Spectrum Disorder[3]
Visual Impairment[4]
Hearing Impairment[5]
Cerebral Palsy[6]

As at January 2012, there are 20 SPED schools and they cater to their target special needs profiles. The list of the 20 SPED schools in Singapore can be found on MOE website and is also stated in Appendix B.

Common issues faced by SPED schools and caregivers in the area of mental health

SPED schools face multiple challenges, the first and foremost being a lack of customised mental health training to meet specialised needs of students. As the special needs sector gains more visibility in the Singapore education scene, the expectation on teachers and allied health professional's services and professionalism has also increased. Often, teachers and allied health professionals in SPED schools have limited practical experience and specialised training in managing mental health issues. Given the complex demands of the children and adolescents they work with, coupled with lack of specialised mental health training, continued professional training to compliment the existing training in other areas is therefore much needed in working with the specific areas of special needs that the school serves. Another challenge is that when training becomes available, SPED school staff find it difficult to find time from their heavy and high demand workloads and lack of suitable relief staff to attend these training.

SPED schools also face difficulties in getting parents to work collaboratively on the behaviours and learning of their children. One of the factors that contribute to this challenge is the lack of appropriate information and education for caregivers on what the special needs entail and how to work in partnerships with other agencies to teach and manage their children. This specific challenge is perpetuated by the lack of social acceptance due to the stigma surrounding people with special needs. These challenges are worsened when coupled with mental health conditions. Such caregivers experience social isolation from their communities, and even from their own family members. Many caregivers experience increased emotional distress, financial hardship, career disruption, social isolation, and worries about their children's future. Some caregivers have revealed that in their efforts to accommodate and focus on their children with special needs, they neglect their other children. These siblings have also voiced their anger and rejection toward their sibling with special needs.

On the other hand, SPED schools also note that some caregivers appear apathetic about the future and well-being of their children. They do not seem to see the need or the inclination to work with the schools early to build consistency in reinforcing and equipping their children with appropriate social and daily living skills. There are also the caregivers who feel helpless in terms of managing the aggressive or inappropriate behaviours of their children at home even after learning the strategies on managing misbehaviours from the school.

For students who require further specialised treatment for their mental health conditions, the allied health professionals do arrange regular meetings with parents and conduct workshops on behaviour intervention and medication within some of the SPED schools. In terms of treatment compliance, the main stumbling block encountered by these allied health professionals is that some caregivers may not be fully aware of or convinced on the efficacy of medication and behaviour intervention. These caregivers often self-medicate or dispense medication to their children as and when they deem it necessary. It is also not uncommon for some caregivers to miss their children's medical appointments, or at times, even stop their follow-ups at clinics.

Consideration for collaboration between REACH and SPED schools

REACH recognised the importance of working with SPED schools as the prevalence of mental health disorders is known to be much higher in children and adolescents with intellectual disability (Dekker & Koot, 2003), Autism Spectrum Disorders (Noterdaeme & Wriedt, 2010), and sensory impairments (Carvill, 2001), compared to the general population. While this appears to be the trend, only a low proportion of these youths with comorbid mental health disorders seek mental healthcare services (Taggart, Cousins, & Milner, 2007).

> *"With REACH successfully implemented in all mainstream schools, it is a natural progression to reach out to the Special Education Schools. REACH will leverage on its five years of experience working with mainstream schools to provide early intervention, support and training to Special Education Schools to improve the mental health of special needs students."*
>
> Dr Daniel Fung, Programme Director (REACH)

On 18 March 2010, a formal dialogue took place to address the availability of resources to SPED school students with mental health concerns. In this meeting, different stakeholders who have been involved in working with children and adolescents with special needs, such as NCSS, MOE, IMH, Health Promotion Board (HPB), and MOH, came together and explored the possibilities for REACH to provide support to the SPED schools. A focus group discussion was also conducted during the dialogue where the SPED schools were divided into four discussion groups based on the special needs type of their students. The four focus groups were: moderate-severe intellectual disability, mild intellectual disability, sensory impairment and Autism Spectrum Disorder, and multiple disabilities. The discussions focused mainly on the common difficulties faced by the schools, services that were lacking, as well as to explore the potential benefits from collaborating with REACH. One of the common responses that came up from all groups was the lack of clear communication between CGC and SPED schools with regard to the diagnosis and follow-up actions with the students during and after treatments. With this in mind, the SPED schools were optimistic that REACH could be the bridge to link CGC and SPED schools more closely. The groups also saw the need for more training in the identification of mental health disorders in SPED school students and to this end, they saw the REACH helpline as potentially being useful in providing appropriate advice and increasing the knowledge of their schools' allied health professionals. Last but not least, the groups also reflected that REACH seems to be a more appropriate channel for increasing caregivers' awareness in the importance of treatment adherence, particularly in the area of medication and behavioural intervention.

Following the formal dialogue, a number of meetings took place between NCSS, MOE, MOH, IMH, and HPB. In those meetings, the multiple stakeholders identified the need and how REACH services can compliment their existing framework. In addition, the group explored the role of each agency and the different expertise and resources they can offer in the implementation of REACH in the SPED schools. A year on from the first formal dialogue, a meeting was held to discuss the objectives of the Project, services provided by REACH, and requirements to the SPED schools to ensure successful collaboration of the REACH-SPED Project.

In summary, the aims of the REACH-SPED Project are as follow:

(1) Provide community mental health services to improve the mental health of the students in the SPED schools;

(2) Develop SPED schools' capacity to detect and manage mental health disorders of students; and

(3) Develop a mental health network for SPED school students in the community.

The ranges of service that REACH can provide are as follow:

(1) Clinical services to students aged 6–18 years old through advice-giving on mental health issues through the REACH helpline;
(2) A responsive evaluation of referred students through the triaging system, and early intervention of child mental health problems;
(3) Train the relevant school personnel in identifying and managing mental health disorders/concerns in their students;
(4) Facilitate networking between schools, social/community agencies, General Practitioner and mental health service providers to better integrate care processes through inter-agency consultations and case conferences.

To help ensure that the objectives of the Project could be better met, REACH proposed several requirements from the SPED schools, which in summary are:

(1) Support of school leaders;
(2) Sharing of SPED school staffs' expertise in their particular special needs type;
(3) Appointment of a liaison person (preferably a psychologist, social worker or counsellor) as referral person and mental health resource person;
(4) Formation of a case management team to support the liaison person;
(5) Time commitment for specialised mental health training;
(6) Completion of assessment forms for referred cases before REACH assessment and 6 months later;
(7) 1- to 2-day attachment at the school for REACH staff for them to understand more in-depth the mental health needs of the SPED students. REACH also encouraged that the appointed liaison person be attached to CGC and/or IMH for learning purposes, although this was optional.

The implementation of REACH services to SPED schools

As mentioned previously, one of the most frequently noted needs from SPED schools was to have training in the identification of mental health disorders. While this can appear straightforward, REACH has noted differences when working with SPED school students as compared to working with mainstream school students. One reason was that students in SPED schools may exhibit symptoms that may be due to their pre-existing conditions, rather than a separate mental health disorder.

> *"The training for Special Educational Schools is different from mainstream schools as certain modules have to be customised to meet the special needs of the student population. These students will require more in-depth mental health assessment as some of the symptoms can be confused with the behaviour caused by their particular conditions."*
>
> Mr Ong Lue Ping, Former Team Leader of REACH South

Thus, a specially tailored series of mental health training programmes was put together by REACH with this in mind. Following the confirmation of the training programs, details were given to NCSS who then disseminated the information to all the SPED schools. The training programmes were the product of the collaborative work between IMH, HPB and NCSS. This took place between July 2011 to October 2011 and was open to all SPED schools.

SPED training topics offered by REACH:

- Mental health issues in children with special needs
- Clinical interviewing
- Conducting mental state examination
- Use of rating scales
- Case formulation
- Working with caregivers of children with mental illness
- Psychopharmacologic treatments

Rounding up the series of SPED mental health training, an overseas expert on dual-diagnosis was invited to Singapore. The visit in Nov 2011 comprise of eight lectures covering key topics raised during the work group meetings and deemed important by the stakeholders. These topics specifically focused on the youth population with special needs from a Canadian perspective. The topics covered were:

(1) Introduction to dual diagnosis;
(2) Behavioural phenotypes and psychological factors associated with genetic syndromes such as Down syndrome and Fragile-X syndrome;
(3) Challenging behaviours;
(4) Issues in identifying Attention Deficit Hyperactivity Disorder, Oppositional Defiant Disorder, and Conduct Disorder;
(5) Assessing for and managing Anxiety Disorders;
(6) Identifying and treating mood disorders;
(7) Psychotic Disorders; and
(8) Psychopharmacology treatments.

REACH helpline and referral service were made available to the four pilot SPED schools in October 2011. The first four SPED schools to access REACH services are MINDS Lee Kong Chian Gardens School, Delta Senior School, Spastic Children's Association School, and Canossian School. These four pilot schools were chosen so that REACH could get a sense of the mental health needs of students with different types of special needs and in different geographical locations of Singapore during the pilot phase. To increase public awareness of the extension of REACH services to SPED schools and the importance of mental health in the special needs population, a media release on this

> *"Working together with REACH to provide a concerted and integrated support system to promote and enhance the social and emotional well-being of our students with special needs, is a long-awaited collaborative project for our school."*
>
> Ms Jacqueline Goh, Psychologist, MINDS Lee Kong Chian Gardens School

project was conducted on 10 October 2011 to coincide with World Mental Health Day.

REACH plans to make the service accessible to all 20 SPED schools by 2013. The tentative plans as of July 2012, was to roll out REACH services to another 7 schools in FY 2012 with approximately two to three SPED schools from each zone, and then roll out REACH services to the remaining 9 schools in FY 2013.

Caregivers and SPED schools' perspective on REACH services

Feedback gathered from the SPED schools and parents have been very positive. In particular, one such feedback was that the REACH team has enhanced the communication and collaboration between SPED schools and mental health professionals by serving as a bridging agency between the schools and CGC. The accessibility of REACH services, as the teams go to schools to conduct the mental health assessments, conferences, and intervention, is deemed as an important feature of the service because parents of SPED schools have additional commitments such as medical appointment and therapies for their children. The accessibility of REACH service is also enhanced through the provision of timely advice and information to parents who may require immediate responses.

Allied health professionals in SPED schools have encountered difficulties in educating parents on the issue of being adherent with treatment. Often, due to the lack of information and appropriate advice on medication, these parents would adjust or stop the medications as and when they deem necessary. On the topic of behaviour management, some parents feel inadequate or disempowered in terms of managing the behaviours of their children which may have deteriorated over the years. Hence, REACH can play an active and crucial role in supporting the SPED schools in the area of caregiver education and training. With regular support from REACH in this area, these parents would be better equipped and have an improved understanding of the role of medications and consistent behaviour management in managing their children's challenging behaviours. Parents could also be in a better position to accept recommendations and be more receptive to working collaboratively with the various stakeholders for their children's overall well-being.

Allied health professionals in the SPED schools lack specialised mental health support services, especially in terms of the difficulties accessing services or trained professionals to seek timely advice and support. With the implementation of REACH for SPED schools, the allied health professionals have reported that they benefited from regular and continued mental health training provided. Moving forward, it is important to conduct systematic research to assess the value of REACH trainings as well as services provided, so as to better cater to the needs of each SPED school in future.

Case study

Kelly is a seventeen years old Indian girl. Her father works as a security guard and her mother is a homemaker and cares for her and her younger brother with Autism Spectrum Disorder (ASD). Kelly's speech development was delayed — she started speaking only when she was three. A quiet child, Kelly was bullied severely when she was studying at a mainstream primary school. Finally, Kelly's difficulties were diagnosed to be the result of a mild intellectual disability and she transferred to a SPED school. However, even in the SPED school, teachers observed that she was quiet, reserved, and usually did not interact with her peers.

Kelly's years in the SPED school passed uneventfully until she was sixteen. The school teachers became worried when they realised Kelly was beginning to cry, talk to herself, and come to school late regularly over several months. At home, her mother observed Kelly to talk and giggle to herself.

Alarmed, the school psychologist referred Kelly to REACH to assess for possible early psychosis. REACH visited Kelly and her mother at their home. During the assessment, it was found that Kelly was preoccupied with an Indian actress. Kelly could not stop thinking of the actress and would be sad if she was kept from watching videos or see photos that featured this actress.

> *After some creative interviewing, Kelly explained the reasons for her talking and giggling to herself. Kelly explained that she was actually asking her favourite Indian actress to come and meet her. She also explained the reason why she came late to school — Kelly often did not have enough sleep because she frequently woke up in the middle of the night as she missed the actress. Kelly's mother reported that Kelly was spending less time watching videos or seeing pictures of this actress after some clear rules were set for her as suggested by the school psychologist. There was no change in Kelly's appetite and she did not seem overtly anxious or depressed.*
>
> *REACH concluded that Kelly did not fulfil the full criteria to warrant an additional psychiatric diagnosis at that point. The odd behaviours observed at home and school, due to Kelly's obsession with the Indian actress, was manageable with some clear rules and did not disrupt her daily functioning. However, the REACH assessors noticed some traits of ASD in Kelly and thereby recommended a plan to support her needs. She was helped to develop prosocial skills, find friends in school, explore her feelings for her favourite actress, and develop her strengths. Parents learned to help Kelly find friends in the community, schedule meaningful activities, and interact more with her. Parents also realised that family harmony could be achieved if they joined support groups which could guide them in dealing with their younger son and his special needs.*

Notes

1. Intellectual Disability is defined as having significant limitations in intellectual functioning and adaptive functioning as expressed in conceptual, social and practical adaptive skills (American Association on Intellectual and Developmental Disabilities. (2010). *Intellectual Disability: Definition, Classification, and Systems of Supports.* Washington DC: AAIDD).
2. Multiple disabilities have two or more impairments, the combination have interactional, rather than additive, effects, making instruction and learning complex. Examples of common Multiple Disabilities include: Cognitive and physical impairments, such as intellectual disability and spastic quadriplegia. Source: Maryland State Department of Education. Retrieved from http://www.mdecgateway.org/olms/data/resource/4797/Multiple%20Disabilities-TA.doc.

3. Autism Spectrum Disorder (ASD) is a neuro-behavioural syndrome resulting from a dysfunction of the central nervous system that leads to disordered development. Source: World Health Organization. (1993). The ICD-10 classification of mental and behavioural disorders: diagnostic criteria for research. Geneva: Author.

4. Visual Impairment, includes both partial sight and blindness, refers to impairment in vision that, even with correction, adversely affects a student's performance. Source: Knoblauch, B. & Sorenson, B. (1998). IDEA's definition of disabilities. In *ERIC Digest* E560. (ERIC Document Reproduction Service No. ED429396).

5. Hearing Impairment is defined as a diminished ability to detect, recognise, discriminate, perceive, and/or comprehend auditory information. Source: New York State Department of Health, Early Intervention Program. (2007). *Clinical Practice Guideline: The Guideline Technical Report.* Hearing Loss, Assessment and Intervention for Young Children (Age 0–3 Years). (Publication No. 4967). New York: Author. Retrieved from http://www.nyhealth.gov/community/infants_children/early_intervention /docs/ guidelines_hearing_loss_recommendations.pdf).

6. Cerebral Palsy refers to a group of disorders of development of movement and posture, causing activity limitations, which are attributed to non-progressive disturbances that occurred in the developing fetal or infant brain. Source: Rosenbaum, P. (2009). Recent Developments in Health Care for Cerebral Palsy: Implications and Opportunities for Orthotics. Denmark: International Society for Prosthetics and Orthotics. Retrieved from http://ispo.web.org.HTML/2009/ispo_cp_report.pdf.

Working with counsellors and MOE psychologists in schools, homes and training events

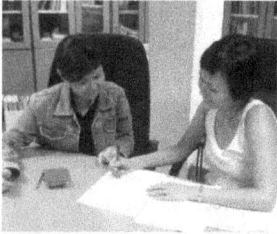

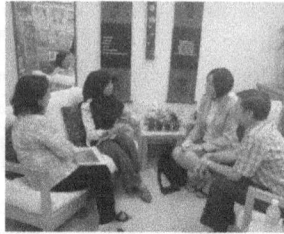

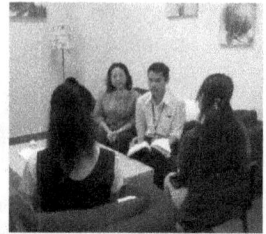

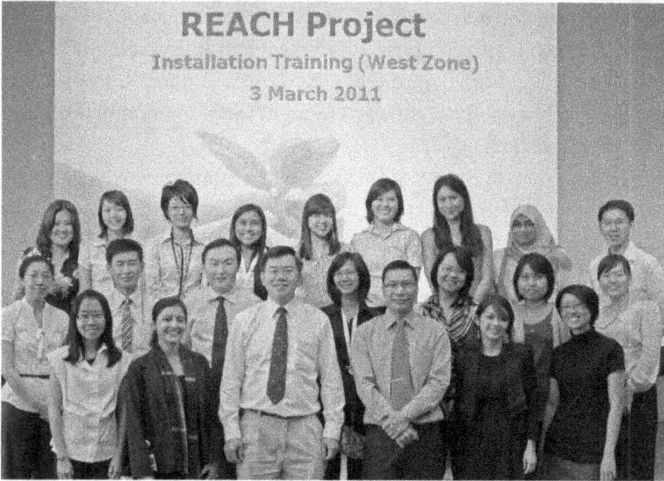

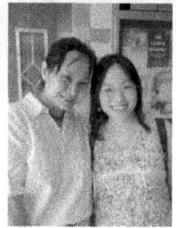

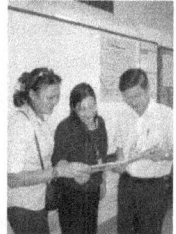

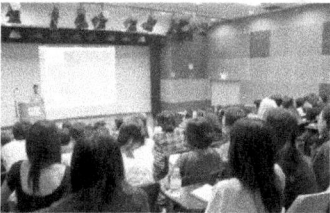

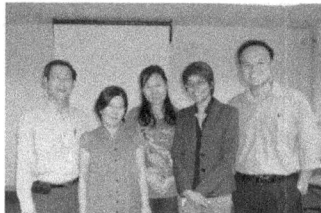

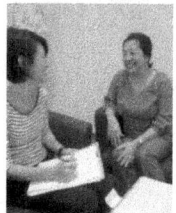

Chapter 4

Partnership with VWOs

Estelle Lim and Liew Shiang Hui

Over time, medical, educational and social systems of care forge partnerships with the communities and the families they come into contact with. While the partnerships can have a positive impact on the delivery and quality of care, these relationships may be strained by different professional understanding and assumptions. This chapter attempts to detail the process involved in developing a collaborative partnership with the intent that others may be able to use a similar framework to start workable positive partnerships with community agencies.

Start with a common reason

VWOs are non-governmental agencies whose main agenda is often about improving the lives of the residents in Singapore. They complement the efforts of government agencies to provide resources to the community. For example, the mentally ill who are abandoned by their families or children who are stateless because the parents are foreigners may need social care and support. VWOs are non-profit organisations which in Singapore are formed in 3 possible ways — as a Society under the Societies Act, or incorporated as a Company Limited by Guarantee under ACRA or formed as a trust. Following their formation as a legal entity under the three options, they can then register for charity status with the Commissioner of Charities.

"A Cochrane review of community-based programmes showed that community team-based psychiatric services led to a reduction in suicide rates, improved patient engagement and were more acceptable to patients."

Tyrer, Coid, Simmonds, Joseph & Marriott, 1999

As part of the mission to reach communities, NCSS provides leadership and directions for VWOs "to ensure that every person has the opportunity to live a life of dignity to his or her fullest potential within society". The development of each VWO is driven by its own vision and mission to serve particular groups in their communities. Their clients however are at times patients of hospitals and students in the schools. Thus collaboration between government related agencies and VWOs is important.

When REACH was being developed, it was clear that besides the school system, VWOs were providing support to schools through a NCSS and MCYS school social work initiative called Enhanced Step Up. Leveraging on this existing framework, a pilot collaboration between REACH and selected VWO partners who work with at–risk youths was initiated.

The Enhanced STEP-UP (School Social Work To Empower Pupils to Utilise their Potential) caters to youth who require additional support and encouragement to remain in school, as well as youth who have already dropped out of school. It is a client-centric school social work programme specifically catered to youth who require additional support and encouragement to remain in school, as well as youth who have already dropped out of the schools. The programme is carried out by participating VWOs, and includes individualised casework, intervention work with the families of the youth, and group activities aimed to support the youth in bringing about positive changes in their lives.

Such a partnership involves two critical roles. Firstly the VWO is the first-line contact of children, youth and families who may be experiencing mental health problems. Some of these students may have dropped out of the school system or are on the verge of dropping out. With the help of the

VWO partner, the student may receive a mental health assessment at home which otherwise may not be done. Secondly, the VWO may also be the best agency to care for the student and their families after a mental health assessment has been carried out.

When REACH started work with schools, some behavioural or emotional problems a student faced were related to family and financial difficulties. The student may want to attend school but have poor coping skills to handle the overwhelming conflicts within their families. For example, with REACH partnership with Beyond Social Services (BSS), one such student is supported with family assessment and counselling and support. Suggestions were made for the student to attend youth appropriate activities at BSS. This helped the student handle the conflicts she had with her family members and improved her school performance as well.

Choosing workable partners

The bio-psychosocial developmental model is used by the REACH team in the evaluation and planning of interventions for youths and their families. This allows the team and the supported school to develop a holistic understanding of the child not just in terms of mental health disorders but the social environment of the child. REACH as a multidisciplinary team with different professional team members take on different intervention tasks. Social workers in the team work on family related issues and become points of contact with VWOs. However, just as each child and their families is different, the VWO who provides care to its clients is also different. Thus in identifying potential partner VWOs, REACH had to first understand their work, their abilities to handle the mental health related work and the additional training required to bridge the gap.

Thornicroft and Tansella (2003) in a WHO Health Evidence Network (HEN) report on community based mental health suggest that the choice of which agencies to partner first depends on traditions and the inclination of agencies to work on mental health, consumer, care giver and professional staff preferences and existing service strengths and weaknesses. A balanced

Table 1. Mental health service components for low-, medium- and high-resource countries

Low-resource countries	Medium-resource countries	High-resource countries
(a) Primary care mental health with specialist backup	(a) Primary care mental health with specialist backup and	(a) Primary care mental health with specialist backup and
	(b) Mainstream mental health care	(b) Mainstream mental health care and
		(c) Specialised/ differentiated mental health services
Screening and assessment by primary care staff	Outpatient/ambulatory clinics	Specialised clinics addressing specific disorders or patient groups, including:
Talking treatments, including counselling and advice		• eating disorders
		• dual diagnoses
Pharmacological treatment		• treatment-resistant affective disorders
		• adolescent services
	Community mental health teams (CMHTs)	Specialised CMHTs, including:
		• early intervention teams
		• assertive community treatment (ACT) teams

approach to community-based mental health services requires a mixed portfolio of services, and the blend depends largely upon the resources available.

Singapore's present capability reflects that she is a medium resourced country moving towards a high resourced country status. The VWOs were identified with the help of NCSS and the pilot group of four, were organisations that were able to take on the additional role of providing mental health services to their clientele. REACH also needed to build a relationship that sought to understand the mission and vision of the VWO, the people who make up the VWO, their culture and how they functioned, their clients, needs, challenges and strengths. The social workers of the REACH teams formed the core team for developing a working relationship with the VWO.

The REACH VWO core team consists of members from REACH North, South, East and West. They meet every quarter to brainstorm ideas and identify training opportunities. In line with resources effectiveness, the VWO core team leverages on the modular training programme developed for school counsellors for the partner VWOs. Like the partnerships with schools, two identified staff members within each VWO partner was necessary as the point person for communication and interface. At the start of discussion the VWO core team members decided in 2010 that academic qualification, work experience and VWO organisational appointment would be the benchmark for the VWO to select their staff for the partnership. The rationale for setting this criteria was that these individuals were to become leaders of mental health awareness in their organisation. They are also expected to train their colleagues within their organisation. Hence, a team member who was more experienced would be a better match to REACH's mandate to not only provide early intervention and assessment, but also in training their organisation and others in the community.

> "I benefited most by gaining more knowledge about how the medical professionals work with each other. This helps me to navigate the system more effectively to help my client in a faster more effective manner. I also feel my agency benefits from being a partner with Child Guidance Clinic as we have quicker access to mental health services."
>
> Dawn, Social Worker, Students Care Service
>
> "I was impressed with the openness of the medical team to other professionals and our viewpoints ...This makes the training beneficial."
>
> Theresa, Social Worker, Students Care Service

In addition to creating processes, a training programme was developed for the VWOs' core team members. The objective of the training was to enhance the capacity of the VWO members to hone their skills in detecting children and youth of at-risk mental health states. The training programme consisted of a lecture series and attachment hours with the Child Guidance Clinic, IMH and the REACH North and South teams. The lecture series

"The intensive clinical training and attachment provided are helpful because we get to learn more about mental illnesses in children and through the attachment, we get a first hand experience observing how the professionals conduct their interventions with the patients."

Jenny Giam, Social Worker, Singapore Children's Society

included equipping VWO professionals with evidence-based assessment tools and knowledge about childhood and adolescent mental health disorders. The attachment with the clinic and community team allowed for clinical experience and provided a platform for case discussion and collaboration of cases where necessary.

Partnership with MOH and NCSS

Another part of the positive partnering was having MOH and NCSS involved in the planning stages. MOH provided the funding while NCSS provided advice on the VWO selection process. NCSS is the statutory body set up to provide leadership and direction in social services, enhance the capabilities of social service organisations, and promote strategic partnerships for social services. NCSS also recommended suitable VWO partners with relevant experience in working with at-risk children and youth. The initial four VWOs selected were The Singapore Children's Society (Yishun FSC), Students Care Service (SCS), Beyond Social Services and MCYC Community Services Society.

NCSS determined in consultation with the VWOs, Key Performance Indicators for reporting and provides usage of the Enhanced Performance Evaluation System, an online system to measure and monitor outcomes for quality assurance. These indicators for the partnership mirror that of the REACH service for schools and GPs.

The long-standing influence of the VWOs' presence in their communities is an asset to the REACH partnership. Many of the clients that are cared for by them are at-risk children and families who are of lower social economic status, and at risk of delinquency and other antisocial behaviours. From pre-launch dialogues with these four VWOs, REACH is able to learn about their work structures and processes to coordinate the provision of services to specific clients.

Our trained VWO partners have first line support from the REACH team through the REACH helpline. The referral process and flow follows that of the School referral to REACH (to be found in chapter 2), where the student's presenting problem will be sorted and prioritised for assessment/advice. After a mental health assessment is carried out, endorsement by the multidisciplinary team and consultant psychiatrist is done, followed by feedback and follow up care for the youth and family in the community. The flexibility of the REACH team allows access to mental health services within the familiar care environment which helps reduce the stigma towards seeking help for mental health issues. In addition, involving a familiar VWO staff that works with the family provides reassurance and support for the youth and family seeking help.

Learning points

One of the key features of a good working partnership between REACH and the VWOs is the recognition that while the organisations are quite similar in their mandates to serve the communities, operations on the ground differs. The approach towards managing a clinical problem and tolerance for atypical behaviours or dysfunctional families varies. This may explain the lower number of referrals from the VWOs to REACH as compared to the schools, although students are still the main clientele. Through reviews and an annual meeting with the VWO leaders and core team members, it is revealed that in some organisations, only certain type of childhood mental health disorders may be encountered. For example in Students Care Service (SCS), many of the children seen are those with academic and financial needs on top of family relationship issues. The staff in SCS may encounter children with ADHD quite often but as the child is attending school and under the purview of the school counsellor, the attention for the child's ADHD management is left to the school. SCS continues with its core service of providing academic support for the child.

VWOs are also found to be highly adept in handling students who drop out of school or who are going through difficult family situations. These students present themselves with emotional issues but with the support of the VWOs, their troubled states do not progress to a clinical level. In this situation, the result is that REACH involvement for assessment may not be necessary.

Since 2010, the partnership has also evolved as the REACH teams understand the needs and barriers better. Openness to change within the year of implementation fostered a positive collaborative partnership and REACH was able to benefit from VWOs' skills and specialisation. A good example is Beyond Social Services who is a leader for advocating community restorative practices. They conducted training for colleagues from REACH and Child Guidance Clinic, about restorative practices. In this workshop, two staff members from Beyond Social Services, provided a 1.5 hours of experiential training on what activities can be used to foster teamwork and trust in teens. Staff from the Child Guidance Clinic were also invited to participate. Most staff had hands-on opportunities and it was an experience that brought fun and laughter.

> "Restorative Practices bring together people when relationships are damaged by the specific actions of one or more people. An effective restorative intervention is one that leads to mutual understanding and an agreed-upon, feasible plan to make things right. A successful restorative process is one in which agreements are kept and relationships are restored—things are made right."
>
> Amos Clifford, 2009

After two years of the partnership, actual referrals to REACH may be small. However, the REACH teams have received more than 100 calls on the helpline and conducted about 30 case conferences for the VWOs. A possible reason is that data collected does not include children and families that VWOs are co-managing with REACH. There is also no tracking of youths who are currently being helped by REACH in schools and are receiving additional support from the VWOs. To date, REACH has trained eight workers from the VWOs as mental health "specialists" within the VWO and setting up the network of mental health support for children in the community. These VWO referred about ten youths and their families to REACH suspected of possibly having emotional disorders like Anxiety Disorder and Depression as well as ADHD. With the partnership, the VWOs are able to plan a more holistic intervention plan for students and families. In addition, the REACH teams have received more than 100 calls on the helpline and conducted about 30 case conferences. The use of REACH as a resource by the VWO partners is encouraging.

> "More staff members to be trained can put stability to the service we provide."
>
> Tan Khye Suan, Executive Director, MCYC Community Services Society

Other initiatives include training and intervention of the Alert programme for ADHD (See Chapter 6) and Anger Management for the Singapore Children's Society's (Yishun FSC). SCS also started an ADHD and mental health awareness weekend in the community, using the resources provided by the partnership. Staff in REACH and community partners have the option to update, consult with and co-service students and their families who may have mental health problems as well as social difficulties.

Extending the partnership beyond the initial four partners

In terms of being able to establish a working network that is sustainable, the VWOs and REACH are in agreement. Journeying ahead, current partnerships have to be deepened to achieve a sense of usefulness while new VWO partnerships need to be developed to widen the network. The next phase of work following consultation with our VWO partners involves customisation of service delivery, workload and case management, while maintaining a similar referral process.

Some other questions that need further brainstorming for a solution would pertain to the nature of referrals. Both VWOs and REACH have to deal with the fine lines of a purely social versus a mental health issue. The timing of intervention and referral for the client and different levels of engagement with the REACH team also require some comprehensive discussion. This is especially crucial when services in the VWOs are chargeable to the client whereas services by REACH are initially free. While costing may be necessary, workers have to be mindful not to have cost become a barrier for clients wanting to receive help.

One of the conceptual plans was for REACH to provide consultative services to VWO partners as they mentor other VWOs interested in this area of work. This could include joint discussions of individual cases seen and also in training sessions and assessments where the REACH team works with the VWO staff. In conjunction with this, REACH was asked to extend the modular training to more staff in the VWO partners. A longer term plan would be research on evidence based community intervention programmes for youths with mental health disorders.

In Oct 2011, Persatuan Persuratan Pemuda Pemudi Melayu (4PM) became a new VWO partner with the REACH programme. 4PM is supported by allowing its staff to join the modular training organised for school counsellors, as well as co-assessment of cases within the community. The extension of training sessions to our VWO and other partners, maximises the use of limited manpower resources. Such cross training also allows networking between participants. REACH seeks to extend its network to 12 VWOs by FY 2013/2014. It is planned that every REACH team will attract at least three VWOs within each of their zones. Location and service rendered may be better matched if that was the case.

The way the VWO network has developed suggests that there is a need for more avenues of training and education in community agencies. This can help to alleviate fears of working with children who are at risk of mental health disorders. The potential influence of an extensive partnership between REACH and VWOs would be reduction of stigma in receiving help for mental health issues in the community. Some families may also have better coping skills if there is accurate detection of a mental health issue and right-siting of care is delivered to the client and their families. The child psychiatric wards in the hospitals may also be providing better care to the most needful child as there could be lesser crowding of hospital beds by children with mental health issues that can be supported within the community. As for the clients, there is a likelihood of lower rates of default for therapy and intervention as VWOs are generally located closer to their homes. At-risk youths are often given that label because of their overt antisocial behaviours and disengagement from school, which could be the result of an underlying mental health problem. Training VWOs to identify mental health disorders benefits youths by directing help to them early, before they go through the school system labelled as a troublemaker and are offered inappropriate interventions targeted at the symptom but not the problem. In worse case scenarios, these youths drop out of the school system and end up in the juvenile justice system as help had not been delivered in a timely and effective manner. All in all, the health of communities can be better served with an extensive, positive working service between VWOs and mental health professionals.

"You address demand first of all by demonstrating that you can make a difference to people's lives when they suffer from these conditions. In any community if you are able to demonstrate impact on individuals, the word gets around."

Professor Vikram Patel, Psychiatrist and former Rhodes Scholar

Training outline for VWO partners

Methods of assessment for the VWO participants during the training are as follows.

A. Evaluation

    a. Baseline evaluation on competency and knowledge in identifying and assessing mental health disorders in children and adolescents

    b. Feedback forms following lectures

B. Individualised Programme

    a. Reflection Log

    b. Clinical Attachment and Clinical Attachment Log

    c. Case presentation

    d. Lecture based Case Discussions

The full clinical training hours and breakdown are as follows.

Full Clinical Training Hours of:

(1) **Lecture Series: 30 hours:** 9 sessions + Introductory lecture + Review session

(2) **Clinical Attachment: 100 hours**

Examples of topics in the lectures conducted in 2010:

- Developmental & Childhood Disorders
- Behaviour Problems & Psychosocial Interventions
- Understanding Psychosis & Schizophrenia
- Clinical Interviewing and Mental State Examination

Clinical Attachment Programme

	Sub total	Total Hours
Clinical Attachment hours		
Psychiatrist Clinic	12	
Psychologist Clinic	12	
Medical Social Worker Clinic	12	
Reach Team Assessment	40	
Sunrise Ward (Child Inpatient Unit)	8	
Neuropsychiatry Clinic	4	
Case Conference Presentation	12	
		100

Participants selected from their VWO organisations were social workers, senior social workers, counsellors, senior counsellors and an executive director. With the end of the training, VWOs officially started referrals to REACH via the REACH Helpline on 1 April 2010. To streamline the referral process, VWOs follow the REACH referral processes with schools (Refer to Chapter 2).

Our VWO partners (2012)

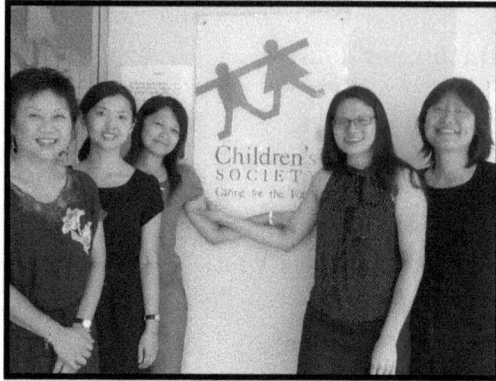

From left: Koh Wah Khoon (Centre Director, Children's Society), Sim Wan Hua (REACH), Jenny Ghiam (Children's Society), Liew Shiang Hui (REACH), & Cheng Pei Yun (Children's Society)

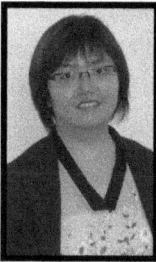

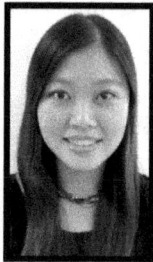

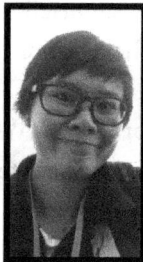

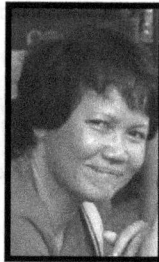

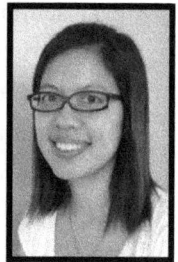

From left: Jennifer Ang-Yeo, Theresa Wang & Ang Kaifen from Students Care Service & Gloria Dom & Lim Shaw Hui from Beyond Social Services.

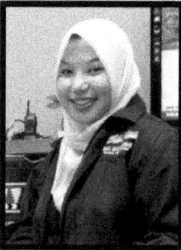

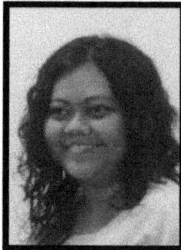

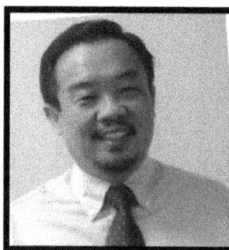

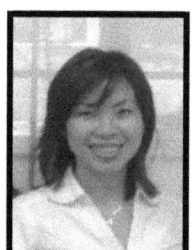

From left: Nadia Bamasari & Evina Subani from 4PM & Tan Khye Suan & Mary Ng from MCYC.

Chapter 5

Partnership with General Practitioners (GPs)

Sim Wan Hua

In recent years, there have been significant changes in the way mental healthcare is delivered to children and adolescents in Singapore. The agenda for these changes was set in 2007 with the implementation of the National Mental Health Blueprint which resulted in a shift in the delivery of care from individual psychiatric institutions to the community. This chapter contains the rationale for mental health management in the community and the vital role played by GPs. Attention is also given to the approach adopted in the planning and implementation of the processes and strategies to optimise the partnership with GPs.

The vision and a GP solution

Mental health disorders are recognised as a public health problem globally, and their management places substantial burden on affected individuals and their families, and increases social and economic costs. According to a report by the World Health Organization (2005), approximately one in five children has a mental health disorder. For parents coping with a child with mental health disorders, the family is directly affected by the mental health system as they try to balance the cost of care and efficient use of resources.

One of the most sustainable responses to meet the increasing demand for mental health services is to implement strategies that can reduce the burden of disease in our community rather than merely provide more care. There is a need to develop and implement strategies for maintaining good mental health as well as those for intervening quickly and effectively when mental health problems occur. In the National Mental Health Blueprint (2007–2012), it was recognised that local healthcare is moving towards a policy of right-siting, where healthcare is dispensed at the appropriate site, thus ensuring better allocation of resources. In particular, the vision is to move away from a hospital-based healthcare delivery system towards a population-based model of mental healthcare.

In Singapore, primary care physicians are commonly known as GPs. According to MOH statistics (Ministry of Health [MOH], 2012), 80% of the primary healthcare services in Singapore are provided by private practitioners. With GPs forming the core of the primary care workforce supporting the healthcare needs of the local population, GPs can play a significant role in detecting and providing primary care services to children and adolescents with mental health problems.

Being the primary care physicians, GPs are often the first point of contact for the majority of children and adolescents. In their practice, GPs have to contend with undifferentiated complaints and symptoms from their young patients and their caregivers who expect them to provide comprehensive and continuing care. Compared to specialist care, GPs are multi-skilled providers and their services are often deemed to be more accessible and convenient. With most GP practices being located in the neighbourhoods, indirect costs associated with seeking healthcare in distant locations are avoided. The provision of after-office hours and weekend consultation times also provide wider options for young patients and their caregivers.

General practitioners also play an integral role of being the main source of healthcare information for patients and their caregivers. Accompanied by a less stigmatising environment, GPs could potentially exercise a strong influence in de-stigmatising mental health conditions and facilitating families' decision-making process with regard to specialised care that may be required for members of the family. Being a steady point of contact for young patients and their caregivers, continuity of care for the optimal management of patients is feasible in general practice as it permits an accessible platform for regular reviews, monitoring of lifestyle changes and co-management of other physical health conditions. Patients with stabilised chronic mental health disorders would also benefit from the relative ease of visiting GPs instead of returning to specialists at the hospitals for regular follow-ups. Moreover, there is enormous potential for GPs to detect, manage and refer patients in the mental health system of care. When the treatment of common mental disorders is integrated into primary care, it can be cost effective and bring important benefits to individuals, families and the society.

GP-School Network

With the initiation of the National Mental Health Blueprint, various community mental health teams and GP Partnerships have been developed to link specialist mental health services with primary care to provide support for different demographic and target groups. To integrate mental healthcare of children and adolescents, a large part of the efforts is channelled to early identification and intervention by the REACH team. This includes engaging the GPs in order to build a network of mental health support for children and adolescents in the community. In conjunction with the relevant ministries, educational and health professionals, the 'GP-School Network' was set up in 2007. The objectives specific to the partnership with GPs include:

i.   To establish a network of GPs for collaborative care between mental health workers & GPs for the management of children and adolescents with mental health disorders.
ii. To increase the capacity of GPs in managing children and adolescents with mental health disorders.

The first objective aims at facilitating links between schools, social service agencies, general practitioners and tertiary mental health service providers. The second objective is related to the desired outcome of having a network of general practitioners who are able to provide value-added,

Benefits of Partnership

"... (it) decreases load on psychiatrists and the mental health system on the whole... also reduces the healthcare burden away from the government.

Dr Peter Lim

Lim, P. (2012, April 4). Personal interview.

"(It) raises the standard of primary care... Parents may feel more comfortable going to GPs... there is less stigma and it is more accessible."

Dr Charity Low

Low, C. (2012, April 3). Personal interview.

affordable, de-stigmatised and convenient care services for children and adolescents.

The GP–School Network is part of the overall national mental health plan to develop a community-based mental health support network for children and adolescents so as to provide right-site of care and to integrate the care processes for improved mental health outcomes. For individuals with mild or stable conditions, being cared for within the community goes a long way both for the patients and the society as improved accessibility of services can also lead to better quality of life while allocating scarce specialist services to those who need them most.

Planning for GP partnership: Implementation framework

To achieve the desired objectives and outcomes set out by the GP–School Network, building a sense of common purpose about what has to change and how they can be changed is the first step in the planning process. In addition, the implementation framework and associated strategies should be realistic and sustainable while being respectful of the context of general practice and maintaining a commitment to a quality system of care.

Receptivity

The aim of the GP-School Network programme is to engage GPs in the detection and management of young patients with mild or chronic mental health disorders based on a sustainable partnership. Hence a large part of the implementation framework is to identify, train and collaborate with a group of GPs who are interested in and willing to manage children and adolescents with mental disorders in the community.

> **Becoming a Partner**
>
> *"It comes down to own motivation and personal altruism and interest...It's a service to the community."*
>
> Dr Peter Lim
>
> Lim, P. (2012, April 4). Personal interview.

As part of its networking strategy, REACH started off recruiting GPs who were in the existing MH-GP Partnership for adults and GPs who already have collaborative relationships with schools in proximity to their practice. Invitations and brochures were sent to GPs across the island, and clinic visits were also conducted to publicise and recruit potential GP partners. A total of 29 GPs have since come on board the partnership.

Supportive infrastructure

For the partnership to be successful, it is essential to ensure that there is sufficient appropriate manpower to manage referrals to GPs, coordinate siting of care and provide other forms of help to GPs where necessary. Under the implementation framework, various strategies are being pursued to attract GPs on board the partnership and to maximise their engagement with the project. Efforts were also made to identify and address barriers to implementation (e.g. skills, resources, costs, incentives, etc).

To enhance work processes, a GP core team was formed within REACH to manage referrals to GP, provide right-site care and manage psychiatric emergencies where needed. Internally, GP partners are assigned to designated REACH team members who will coordinate the referral and care for individual patients in the programme. This allows closer monitoring of cases under the care of GPs as well as facilitating the development of working relationships between REACH and GPs.

Besides having a comprehensive professional development programme for GPs, of equal importance to highlight is the development of a seamless drug management and delivery system. At the very least, the system has to ensure that the costs of medication to GPs are kept low so that the final cost charged to patients at the GP clinics would be comparable to that offered at the hospitals. To achieve this, Child Guidance Clinic (CGC) negotiated with key pharmaceutical companies to extend the discounts offered to IMH to the GP partners. This arrangement allows GP partners greater flexibility in pricing their services with concurrent guidelines provided by CGC.

Strategies to improve GP engagement:

1. Clarity in practice policies and standing protocols regarding the referral workflow, use of drugs, case monitoring and commitment to training for GPs
2. Procurement of medications at prices comparable to that of hospitals
3. Flexibility in charging patients with proposed guidelines from Child Guidance Clinic
4. Availability of opportunities for professional development
5. Direct access for consultation with psychiatrists at the hospitals
6. Support in care management by REACH

Capacity building

Critical to the process of developing and implementing the partnership is enhancing the capacity of GPs to detect and manage child mental health conditions. Following a focus group conducted under the existing IMH-GP partnership programme to identify the training needs of GPs in child mental health, a training programme for GPs was drawn up so that they could obtain the skills and knowledge required to support children and adolescents. The training programme comprises group training and seminars on specific child mental health conditions, as well as GP specific training through clinical attachments, case discussions and live supervisions coordinated by CGC. The mandatory component of the training for GP partners includes two live supervisions and six hours of clinical attachment. By offering means of observation, modeling and immediate feedback, live supervisions and clinical attachments provide clinicians with opportunities to develop their skills while monitoring treatment.

A milestone in local psychiatric training was achieved when the Graduate Diploma in Mental Health (GDMH) was launched in 2010 with the joint efforts of the National University of Singapore and IMH to provide a one-year course for GPs in psychiatry and counselling (Institute of Mental Health, 2011). The GDMH aims to provide a comprehensive and structured training programme for GPs to equip them with skills and knowledge for their role in community mental health care. The six-module course covers a segment dedicated to child and adolescent mental health which includes learning disabilities. Another effort towards preparing doctors in community mental healthcare is the Family Medicine training programme which will now include a core posting in psychiatry as part of the training for aspiring doctors who want to become GPs. Both programmes support the Mental Health Blueprint which emphasises the strengthening of mental health

---

What was Helpful for GPs

"REACH gives good support to GPs. Psychiatrists (from IMH) are also easy to reach for consultations for complex cases."

Dr Charity Low

Low, C. (2012, April 3). Personal interview.

"I've found the usual lectures, tutorials, and sit in with psychiatrists at IMH to be helpful and sufficient."

Dr Peter Lim

Lim, P. (2012, April 4). Personal interview.

manpower and appropriate provision of mental health services within the community. To date, six of our REACH-GP partners have enrolled and graduated from the Graduate Diploma in Mental Health programme.

Patient-centric and whole of population approach

The GP partnership is formed based on the principles of a patient-centric and whole of population approach to care. A patient-centric approach means that the patient is actively involved in decision-making and is cared for in a holistic manner by GPs and other mental health workers where required. In adopting a population approach to care, the partnership should identify and target all patients eligible for care by GPs.

Since its conception in 2007, the REACH team has been working with GPs to manage children and adolescents with common mental health disorders such as ADHD. Following the right-siting of care approach, one of the eventual goals of the GP-School Network Programme is for schools to identify and refer at-risk children directly to GPs for diagnosis and treatment.

In the initial phase of the partnership, referrals received by the REACH team are being screened for suitability for assessment and management by GPs. Those that are identified to be suitable are being followed up by a member from the team to contact patients and their families to consult on the recommended siting of care and associated charges. With the assistance of a REACH member, caregivers of young patients select the clinic of a participating GP. Patients and caregivers who are willing to pay the difference in price for the convenience of right-sited care are then assisted by the team to make the first appointment with the GP. Patients with stabilised conditions may also be screened and referred by specialists to GPs where deemed appropriate. To ensure a seamless transition of care to the GP, a designated care coordinator from the REACH team helps in coordinating all aspects of the transfer of care.

To increase patient's involvement in their own healthcare, GPs also explore the social circumstances and barriers that patients face during the consultation (e.g., financial difficulty, family issues). Some GPs have provided help by enlisting support from other health professionals or linking up the patients with community resources such as the VWOs and patient support groups. Other GPs have exercised great flexibility to suit the financial circumstances of families, including that of charging patients lower consultation fees and providing a prescription while patients purchase the medication at the hospital which has lower medication fees due to the economies of scale. In the event that specialist services are needed, GPs could also refer patients for tertiary care provided at the hospital. As the project matures, with the enhanced capacity of teachers and counsellors in identification of mental health problems in children, direct referrals are made from schools to GPs for diagnosis and management. The challenge for the GP is to balance the expectations of patients and schools to provide comprehensive services while ensuring best practice of care for the individual.

Early Challenges Reported by GPs

- Making a confident diagnosis of mental health disorders in children and adolescents
- Managing side-effects of psychotropic medicine
- Deciding on the type, brand and amount of psychotropic medicine to procure and dispense
- Sorting out the cost-effectiveness of procuring psychotropic medicine
- Handling the lack of communication from schools for the management of patients
- Dealing with differences in consultation time for psychiatric versus non-psychiatric patients

Reviewing and adapting implementation

The model of the partnership was developed over time. Periodic reviews on the implementation of the GP-School Network provide opportunities for reflection, adaptation and development of strategies for improvement. The key part of the improvement process is to assess whether the various implementation strategies are enhancing the access, delivery and uptake of mental health services. While the GP's relationship with his or her patient is likely to continue over time, the strategies for care may change such as when patients return to or are referred for specialist care due to changes in their health conditions. As such, some form of measurement is necessary to provide an accurate indication of progress. A number of process and outcome key performance indicators were formulated to measure the effectiveness of the GP programme and have to be reported to MOH periodically.

In line with the objective of establishing a GP network, the programme has successfully partnered 29 GPs and referred 69 patients from schools and 46 patients from IMH to GP care to date. With regard to the objective of providing training to GPs on managing mental health conditions, 223 GPs have attended at least one training session to date. More than 90% of GPs who have attended the training sessions reported satisfaction with the training content and delivery.

Improved mental health of children and adolescents in school is the desired outcome of the community partnership programme. This is being monitored and evaluated by measuring improvement in assessment scores by GPs on the Children's Global Assessment Scale (CGAS) and the Clinical Global Impression (CGI) scale. Further outcomes are expected to be developed as the partnership progresses and expands across the island. Elaboration on the KPIs related to GP partnership can be found in Chapter 7: Taking Stock and REACHing Beyond.

Satisfaction with Partnership

Improved access and provision of mental health services were identified as the key objectives of the National Mental Health Plan for Children and Adolescents. The co-location of a zonal REACH team and specialist services within the vicinity of the general practice was first piloted as a model of service delivery in the North zone and then extended to other regions of Singapore. Benefits expressed by GPs include increased confidence in managing patients with mental health problems, support in overcoming difficulties, and easy access to psychiatrists for support. Since 2008, more than eighty percent of parents of students reported being satisfied with the coordination of care to GPs and the plan of care communicated by GPs.

Continuing challenges

The management of people with mental health problems in general practice presents a number of difficulties. For community mental healthcare to succeed, the implementation of the GP programme should be systematic and whole of practice oriented. This involves a shift in perspective for many practitioners who are used to focusing on individual patients and their acute needs due to their primary training in family medicine. Some of the continual challenges perceived by GP partners in managing young patients with mental disorders include extended consultation time, high default rates, personal or parental preference for treatment by other non-medicine modalities, and skills and knowledge in managing co-morbid psychiatric disorders. The enlisting of GPs on board the partnership is further hindered by the belief that psychiatric illnesses are difficult to manage in general practice and the associated unwillingness of individual GPs in taking responsibility for primary psychiatric care.

On the other hand, the expansion from five GPs during the pilot phase to the current total of 29 GPs has also put pressure on the programme and necessitated the REACH team to ensure that GP partners obtain referrals so as to sustain their interest and capability in managing mental health disorders in the community. At present, the proportion of people with mental health disorders that are being attended to in their practice still constitutes a relatively small proportion. Despite efforts to right-site the care to the community, a substantial number of parents rejected referrals to management in general practice. One of the reasons cited by parents is their preference for care at a specialist centre due to its comprehensive and multidisciplinary care services. Other reasons that were mentioned are related to higher costs and unavailability of non-standard drugs at some GP clinics.

Future directions

While specialist mental health services will never be able to meet the steady demand for treatment on their own, general practitioners are well placed to provide accessible mental healthcare to the majority. The GP-School

Network programme, heralded by the National Mental Health Blueprint and the launch of REACH, has helped create community awareness on mental health issues in school aged children and adolescents. Proactive actions taken by the REACH team since the inception of the programme helped to weather challenges along the way. However, certain perceptions and challenges remain and may deter GPs from partnering in the programme. Continuing community education is needed to reduce stigma and encourage people to seek healthcare for mental health problems.

Ongoing Efforts Necessary

- Raising public awareness of mental health as an integral part of general health

- Building primary care capacity in detecting and treating mental health disorders

- Recruiting more GPs in the integrated care model

It is envisioned that over time, general practitioners will become more confident and proficient in managing mental health problems in the community. The Graduate Diploma in Mental Health jointly managed by the National University of Singapore and IMH is one of recent concerted efforts towards strengthening primary mental healthcare. It is hoped that the treatment of mental health problems will ultimately be comparable to that of physical health conditions, with general practitioners providing most of the ongoing care while being supported by specialist mental health services. The journey towards integrated mental health care will be long, but one that will lead to improved access to services, better quality of life for young people and their families while de-stigmatising mental health disorders in society.

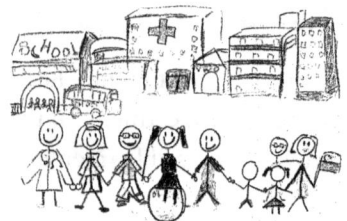

About the GPs cited in this chapter

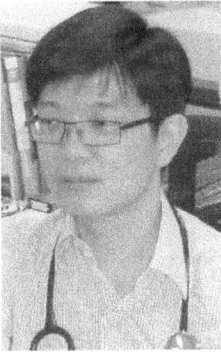

Dr Peter Lim Khoon Boon is a general practitioner with his own practice at Joash Family Clinic and Surgery. He completed his medical training in 1992 at the National University of Singapore (MBBS) and served in the hospitals for the Ministry of Health until 1998. Subsequently, Dr Lim has been serving the community in private practice. While his main area of training and experience is in Dermatology, he has an active interest in mental illnesses and child behavioural disorders.

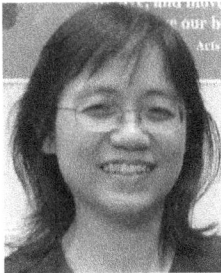

Dr Charity Low Cheng Hong is a senior Family Physician with her own practice at Woodlands, Peace Family Clinic. She graduated from the medical school at the National University of Singapore in 1994. She obtained her masters in Family Medicine in 2006 and the Graduate Diploma in Family Practice Dermatology in 2007, and was admitted as a Fellow into the College of Family Physician Singapore in 2011. Dedicated to teaching and inspiring students with vision and passion for medicine, she holds clinical teaching and tutoring positions in NUS Yong Loo Lin Medical School and Duke-NUS Graduate Medical School. Her personal interests are reading and cooking.

Dr Low has a special interest in Mental Health, Dermatology and clinic procedures and minor surgeries. She is one of the pioneering general practitioners recruited under the REACH programme to manage ADHD children in the community. Currently, she is also a member of the workgroup committee for the upcoming ADHD Clinical Practice Guidelines, an effort to standardise ADHD management locally with reference to the best available scientific evidence and to promote awareness of this prevalent condition in healthcare professionals. In collaboration with IMH, she had completed a research project validating PHQ-9 and QIDS-SR$_{16}$ as valid and reliable screening tools for depression in busy local primary care clinic, contributing insight to the local scene on depression.

Resources

July Lies

REACH resource for intervention			
Tapping programmes & services from CGC	**Programmes to meet the rising needs**	**Using IT as bridge to community**	**Linking up with internal programmes & services**
Meeky Mouse Programme	CyberWiz	Roc-N-Ash Web Portal	LYRIKS
Kucinta Cat Programme		REACH website	SASSI
Alert Programme			
Anger Management Programme			
Incredible Years® School Age Programme for Parents			
Future programmes & services	*Future programmes & services*	*Future programmes & services*	*Future programmes & services*

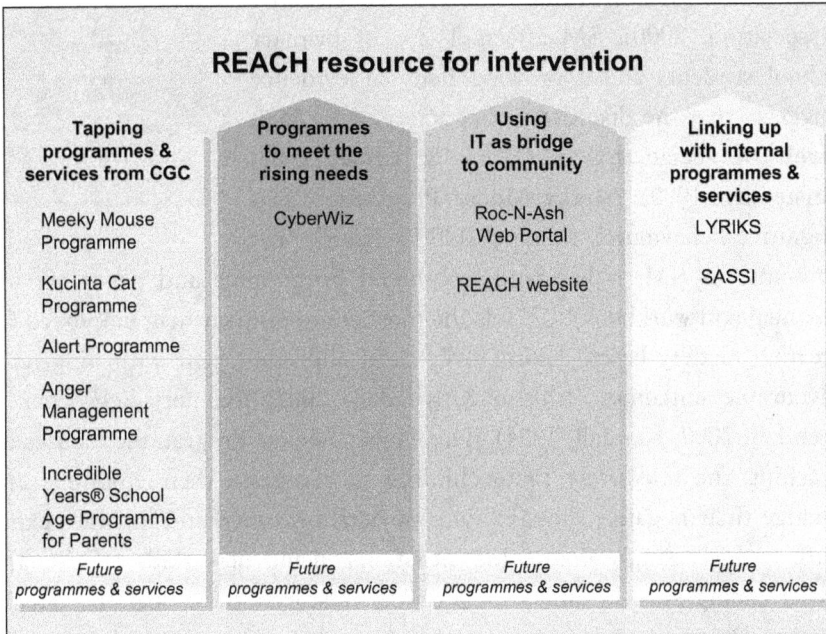

Upon the completion of assessment and case conference, some cases that require intensive treatment will be referred back to the Child Guidance Clinic (CGC) and some cases that would benefit from brief treatment are managed in the school. For the latter cases, REACH team member and school personnel (usually the school counsellor) collaboratively carry out treatment (i.e., programme and services) in the school. This chapter looks into these different treatments provided in school, which are divided into four categories.

Tapping on programmes and services from the Clinic Guidance Clinic

Meeky Mouse Programme

Selective Mutism (SM) is a childhood disorder defined as a lack of speech in selected social settings despite fluent speech in others (American Psychiatric Association, 2000). SM affects 1–2% of primary school students and a growing body of evidence suggests that the disorder is characterised by high levels of social anxiety (Black & Uhde, 1995; Anstendig, 1999). Meeky Mouse Programme is a cognitive-behavioural therapy (CBT) based programme for SM, it has both web-based programme and paper version (manual and workbook). CBT is the most common treatment employed for treating anxiety-based disorders in child and adolescent with long-term favourable outcomes (Albano & Kendall, 2002; Flannery-Schroeder & Kendall, 2000; Kendall, 1994). The Meeky Mouse Programme focuses on teaching the selectively mute children to recognise their emotions and change their negative thoughts in a proactive manner, and includes exposure to increasingly distressing situations, using new skills taught, and experiencing success and self- rewards. Research show that the Meeky Mouse Programme is more suitable for selectively mute children with predominantly anxiety symptoms, aged between 8–12 years, English-speaking and with active parents involvement (Fung, Manassis, Kenny & Fiksenbaum, 2002).

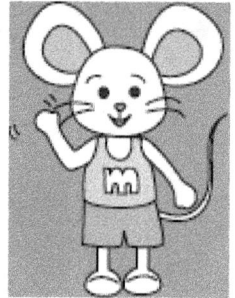

The 14-week Meeky Mouse Programme consists of eight training and psychoeducation sessions followed by six practice sessions (exposure using social skills training). In the eight sessions of skills teaching, the child learns to recognise and identify negative thoughts, feelings, physiological symptoms of anxiety, using the CHAT Plan:

- Check out how my body is feeling (recognising and identifying feelings, physiological symptoms of anxiety, teaching relaxation)
- Having bad thoughts (identifying negative thoughts, self-talk)
- Attitudes and actions that help (brave talk, alternative thoughts and actions)
- Time for reward

The six practice sessions focus on putting skills learned into practice, where the child learn to apply skills (i.e., CHAT Plan) in different situations and social settings, such as building confidence, understanding people, making friends, keeping friends, and handling difficult situations.

REACH provide trainings to school counsellor on the web-based Meeky Mouse Programme and conducts this intervention together with the school counsellor in the school for students with SM. Both the web-based programme and paper version include materials for parents and teachers. Parents can access the manual to help them become more familiar with SM and the intervention plan that targets their child's symptoms of anxiety and selective mutism. Parents will work with their child's therapist in putting the plan to action and are encouraged to work with their children on their homework. In addition, parents can access The Quiet Room, a page devoted to helping parents find resources and help for their children with SM. A set of materials for parents and teachers are available at http://www.imh.com.sg/Quietroom.

Implementing the Meeky Mouse Programme in the school, REACH facilitates close collaboration between school, parents and therapist in helping student with SM. Indirectly, through the use of the Meeky Mouse Programme, school counsellors also benefit from learning how to help children with SM. As most students with SM do not speak in school, it is important to involve the school in the treatment plan as well. Parents are given suggestions on how they can collaborate with the school in helping their children. The ability of REACH to work with student directly in school enhances collaborative efforts and enables these students to apply skills learnt in the real school setting. Conducting the treatment in familiar school environment helps to reduce their initial anxiety and build rapport. Some students may be more comfortable working with school counsellors whom they are familiar with. Moreover, web-based programme may be particularly useful in the treatment of children with SM because it reduces interaction with the therapist through increased interface with the computer. This strategy can be used to help the child to be more at ease in receiving treatment during the initial sessions.

Kucinta Cat Programme

In recent years, CGC has seen an increase in the number of anxiety cases. Anxiety is one of the most common mental health conditions in childhood and research shows the prevalence is as high as 10% (APA, 2000). As mentioned previously, CBT is currently the most empirically-validated treatment for childhood anxiety (Albano & Kendall, 2002; Flannery-Schroeder & Kendall, 2000; Kendall, 1994). "Kucinta Cat" is a CBT based treatment, used in CGC, targeting child and adolescent with anxiety disorder. Kucinta Cat was adapted from Philip C. Kendall's The Coping Cat Programme by CGC psychologists to make it more relevant to the local context. For child and adolescent with anxiety disorder, CBT is usually the first line of treatment and medications are generally not recommended, except for severe cases. Hence, for child and adolescent with anxiety traits/disorders who do not need medications, REACH would carry out Kucinta Cat programme collaboratively with school counsellor in school.

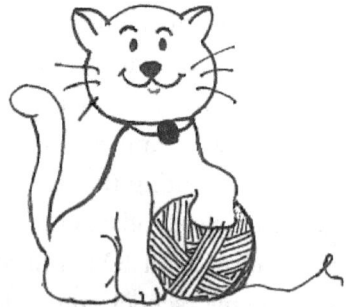

Kucinta Cat programme is an eight-session anxiety management programme taught in a developmentally appropriate manner to upper primary school students. Kucinta Cat is conducted with a standard workbook and includes a parent component. In this programme, children learn to identify feelings and bodily symptoms of anxiety and how to deal with anxiety-provoking situations through various strategies. The programme focuses on four related components:

- Recognising anxious feelings and physical reactions to anxiety
- Clarifying feelings in anxiety-provoking situations
- Developing a coping plan (e.g. coping self-talk, deep breathing)
- Evaluating performance and administering self-reinforcement.

Show That I Can (STIC) tasks are homework exercises that allow children to practise the skills outside therapy sessions. Points are awarded for completed tasks and can be exchanged for rewards.

REACH psychologists who have used Kucinta Cat Programme in school find it easy to implement and students generally have little difficulty understanding the concepts and skills taught. Parents also find the psych-oeducational materials very useful in helping them understand their children better and learning how to respond appropriately to their children's anxiety. School counsellors have observed improvements in some of these students and they are highly encouraged to act as co-therapist during the sessions so they can also benefit from learning basic anxiety management techniques which they can then use to teach other anxious students. The use of Kucinta Cat Programme in school thus reduces the need for referral to CGC, enables students displaying anxious traits to receive early interventions conveniently in the community, and also enhances the knowledge and skills of school counsellors in managing students with anxiety in school.

Alert Programme

REACH has been receiving referrals for ADHD, or students with inattention difficulties. These students have difficulties in paying attention in school and at home, and are often raised as concerns of teachers and parents. Researchers have noticed association between ADHD and sensory integrative dysfunctions (Dunn & Bennett, 2002; Mangeot *et al*, 2001; Parush *et al*, 1997; Smith–Roley, Blanche & Schaaf, 2001). This means that child and adolescent with ADHD may have difficulties with sensory integration. In addition, there are also children and adolescents who do have sensory integration dysfunction without ADHD and have difficulties in sustaining attention.

The Alert Programme® uses the principles of sensory integration to help individuals regulate their alertness level to meet situational demands. This programme was developed by Mary Sue Williams and Sherry Shellenberger, and can be used with pre-schoolers, school students and even for adults. Occupational therapists in CGC have been conducting the Alert Programme® in the clinic and REACH has decided to offer the service to those students with ADHD or who have difficulty regulating their alertness level.

The group runs for approximately about six to ten weekly sessions, together with the school counsellor and another REACH team member. Each group has between four and ten students. The structure of the sessions is as follows:

- Students learn on awareness of their own engine level.
- Students experiment with various sensory strategies, namely tools for eyes, ears, mouth, body/hands.
- Students will determine which sensory strategy helps them.
- Students consolidate what they have learnt and use problem solving skills to apply the sensory strategies in various settings.
- Parents are encouraged to attend the first and last sessions so as to allow them to understand their child's preference of sensory strategies to help them regulate their alertness level.

As of February 2012, REACH from the North, South and East zone has run the Alert Programme with two VWO partners, two primary schools and two secondary schools. Some information on the Alert Programme and the collaboration with VWO partners can also be found in Chapter 4. REACH occupational therapists have also conducted a series of workshops for school counsellors on how strategies of the Alert Programme® can be used with students in schools. These workshops have received overwhelming responses and school counsellors expressed high satisfaction. For that reason, the Alert Programme® and the strategies have been well received by school counsellors, teachers, parents and students. Occupational therapists hope to continue to run this programme so that students with ADHD and inattention difficulties can benefit from the strategies shared from the Alert Programme®.

Case study

As a ten year old, Sam was familiar with being scolded by teachers and adults for various activities. He was constantly on the move, and got into trouble so quickly, he was beginning to suspect that his middle name was Trouble.

REACH came into the picture when the teachers decided that his difficulties in following instructions and focusing in class was not normal for his age. Sam was relieved when REACH told him that he had attention deficit hyperactivity disorder (ADHD) and that there were ways he could help himself to cope.

The REACH occupational therapist conducted nine group sessions of a special programme known as the ALERT programme in Sam's school, with the support of the school counsellor. During these sessions, Sam learnt to identify his "engine levels" when he was in various situations. He figured out how he could use various strategies on different parts of his body to modulate his "engine levels."

For instance, Sam identified that his "engine level" becomes high after recess when he returns to class and talks to his friend. To help modulate his energy levels, Sam decided that he could use one of several strategies: either to drink a cold drink during recess, help teacher clean the whiteboard, or fidget with keychains to calm himself and bring his engine to just the right level. Sam's parents also learnt strategies to apply at home. The REACH occupational therapist also continued to work with the school counsellor to implement Sam's ideintified strategies into the classroom.

After these sessions, the school counsellor gave feedback that Sam was more able to cope and focus and she was very keen to try out the strategies in classroom settings. The school counsellor was also more confident in managing his classroom behaviours with visual cue cards and stories in which Sam have identified helpful for him. In additional, school counsellor found the strategies helpful for herself and her work with students.

Anger Management Group

In some of the cases referred to REACH, the school identified the student to have significant anger as a behavioural difficulty, in addition to his or her diagnosis. REACH offer the Anger Management Group to equip school counsellors with skills to manage students with anger issues in group setting by using the material "Helping Angry Children and Youth Strategies that Work" by Dr Rebecca Ang and Dr Ooi Yoon Phaik. The training programme focuses on teaching the student problem-solving and social skills which are essential life-skills for children to acquire to become socially responsible adults. It is essential that student learn to manage and regulate their emotions, communicate with others effectively and possess positive coping strategies to handle conflict successfully. Some students seem to be constantly angry — they struggle with behavioural difficulties as demonstrated by defiance, fighting, cursing, and name-calling. The strategies and activities presented in this manual, and the workbook are particularly helpful for children with behavioural problems (Ang & Ooi, 2003). A parent training manual called "Seeing Red" is also available for parents (Fung & Ang 2006).

REACH provide the Anger Management Group when it is requested by the school counsellor. REACH team member and school counsellor would discuss the target group between four to eight students. There is a total of eight sessions of anger management and they cover the following materials:

- Identification of feelings
- Exploring anger feelings
- Anger coping techniques I & II
- Perspective-taking and empathy
- Problem-solving skills
- Fighting fair
- Prosocial skills

Schools which had gone through the programme gave very positive feedback with regards to the outcome. "No more complaints from the form teachers after lesson 4" a school counsellor feedback. Parents were pleased with the results too. "There were fewer calls from the school complaining about the child's behaviour" a parent commented.

Incredible Years® School Age Programme for Parents

Parents play an imperative role in the development of their child, and very often, children become the bearer of symptoms in the family; be it due to dysfunctional family dynamics, lack of parental attention, or parenting skills deficit. The Incredible Years® Series — developed by Dr. Carolyn Webster-Stratton, Professor and Director of the Parenting Clinic at the University of Washington — are research-based, and proven effective programmes for reducing children's aggression and behaviour problems and increasing social competence at home and at school. The training programmes give parents strategies to manage behaviours such as aggressiveness, ongoing tantrums, and acting out behaviors such as swearing, yelling, hitting and kicking, answering back, and refusing to follow rules.

The short-term goals of the Incredible Years® Series are to:

- Strengthen children's social skills and appropriate play skills (turn taking, waiting, asking, sharing, helping, complimenting).
- Promote children's use of self-control strategies such as effective problem solving steps.
- Increase emotional awareness by labeling feelings, recognising the differing views of one-self and others and enhancing perspective taking.
- Boost academic success, reading and school readiness.
- Reduce defiance, aggressive behavior, and related conduct problems such as noncompliance, peer aggression and rejection, bullying, stealing and lying.
- Decrease children's negative cognitive attributions and conflict management approaches.
- Increase self-esteem and self-confidence.

REACH (West) is currently conducting a pilot run of the Incredible Years® School Age Programme for Parents in order to better support parents and equip them with parenting skills. The Pilot Programme commenced in March 2012, and spans across 12 weekly sessions. The group consists of nine parents from seven families, who are parenting children from 7–12 years old. Through the programme, parents learn new ideas and methods to help improve their child's behaviour. The group also serves as a safe setting for parents to share the challenges that they face in parenting, and to collaboratively generate solutions to their challenges. The programme contents are as below:

Session 1: Welcome and introduction to programme parents' goal
Session 2: Importance of parental attention and special time
Session 3: Social, emotion and persistence coaching
Session 4: Social, emotion and persistence coaching
Session 5: Effective praise and encouragement
Session 6: Using tangible reward programmes to motivate your child
Session 7: Rules, responsibilities and routines
Session 8: Predictable learning routines and clear limit setting
Session 9: Ignoring misbehaviour
Session 10: Time out to calm down
Session 11: Time out to calm down
Session 12: Other consequences, review and celebration

Parents in the pilot programme have given positive feedback thus far, rating effectiveness of the programme at 97% (percentage is an average obtained from weekly evaluation forms given to parents after every session). They have also shared that they appreciate the positive friendship and support formed over the sessions. With the encouraging feedback, REACH (West) will be continuing with the programme. The next run of the Incredible Years® School Age Programme for Parents is stipulated to commence in August 2012.

Programme to meet the rising needs

Cyber Wellness in the Z-generation (CyberWiz)

REACH received many calls from the school counsellors with regards to students being involved with excessive computer usage (ECU) resulting in sleeping in class, deterioration in school results, family and social issues and school refusal. A local research was done to study the prevalence of exces-

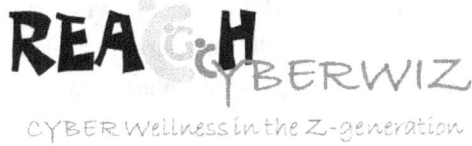

REA·H CYBERWIZ

CYBER Wellness in the Z-generation

sive computer usage among youth. The research was conducted on 2735 adolescents and the result shows that while a quarter of the adolescents surveyed reported that they did not access the Internet everyday, a significant number (17.1%) of adolescents reported using it for more than five hours every day (Mythily, Qiu & Winslow, 2008).

Recognising the need surfaced from the schools and significant prevalence of ECU in Singapore, REACH decided to develop a programme to support the school, the students and the family. After many months of discussion and meetings and gathering manpower and participants, Cyber Wellness In the Z-generation (CyberWiz) was developed and started its pilot project on Dec 2009.

CyberWiz is a three-and-a-half-day day camp for adolescent with ECU. The distinguishing feature of CyberWiz is its inclusion of specific parent-focused and parent-inclusive programmes to complement the acquisition of new skills and practice sessions for the student participants. Parents will be given specific training on the management of their child's ECU issues while combined parent-child (joint) sessions will serve as a forum for students and their parents to learn how to cope and manage ECU issues together through creative and interactive modules and activities.

REACH has organised a total of three CyberWiz camps during the school holidays. Besides creating awareness of ECU, the camps were structured to get participants to start thinking about change, to improve parent-child relationship, to equip themselves with the means to break free from computer dependency and to be able to eventually reintegrate into the real world.

For the first two camps, all facilitators were staff from the REACH programme from IMH. For the last CyberWiz camp, three volunteer staff from Covenant Family Service Centre co-facilitated with REACH in running the camp. The CyberWiz core team also ran monthly support groups with parents and adolescents who had participated in the camps. These support groups allowed parents a platform to share their experiences and gave them a safe environment to talk about their challenges at home and to encourage and affirm other parents.

Questionnaires were given to participants after the camps to gauge the effectiveness of the sessions and camps in raising awareness of ECU and managing ECU. As a whole, the camps received positive feedback from both the adolescent and parents who attended the camps. Data from measures looking at problematic computer usage and parent-child relationships indicated that CyberWiz has been effective in meeting its objectives. Both adolescent and parents reflect that the intensity of problematic internet usage decreased six months after the camp. In addition, both the parent and teen indicated that both parents and adolescent were more satisfied with their relationship with each other.

Going forward, adolescents with ECU will be referred to the National Addition Management Services (NAMS). NAMS offers the adolescent clinic to teenagers between 13 to 19 years old with problems pertaining to ECU, gambling, and substance abuse. Referrals can be made by parents, schools, polyclinics, MCYS, and any relevant agencies.

In terms of looking at benefits of CyberWiz, it created another opportunity for REACH to collaborate and partner with community resources, thus strengthening REACH's networking relationship with other voluntary welfare organisations (VWOs). School counsellor feedback that CyberWiz was a useful source of help they can turn to. They found it to be an intensive programme, and appreciate the speciality in the area of addiction which they are not confident in handling.

Using IT as bridge to community

Reaching Out to Children N Adolescents at School and Homes (Roc-N-Ash) Web Portal

ADHD and Anxiety disorders are two of the most common mental health disorders commonly seen at CGC. However, due to limited resources, there is often a long wait-time before the students with these disorders receive treatment. Hence, Reaching Out to Children N Adolescents at School and Homes (ROC-N-ASH, http://www.roc-n-ash.com) was developed as part of the solution to provide early intervention to the child and adolescent with ADHD and/or Anxiety disorders in the community.

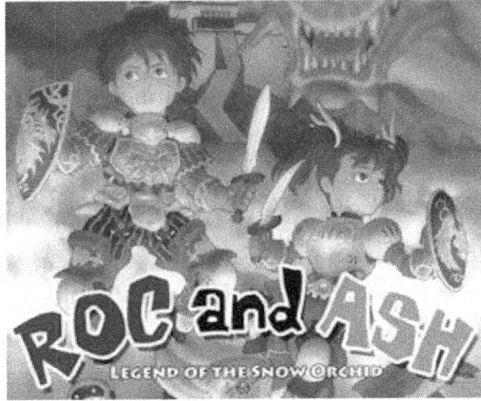

ROC-N-ASH involves a tripartite collaboration between Mental Health Professionals, Infocomm Experts and e-Learning/Gaming Professionals. It was developed as an innovative and holistic IT system to manage the mental wellness of the child and adolescent. ROC-N-ASH enables healthcare professionals to leverage on the system to promote mental wellness of the child and adolescent and facilitate early detection and intervention for children with mental health disorders. It also encourages the involvement of MOE, schools and caregivers to support the management of child and adolescent with mental health disorders.

The ROC-N-ASH portal is an interactive system with information courseware on ADHD and Childhood Anxiety Disorder, Books Purchase/Events Announcements and Therapeutic Games. The information courseware is free for public use and aims to increase public knowledge of ADHD and Anxiety disorders and provide strategies on managing child and adolescent with such disorders. Public can also purchase mental health related books, be informed of upcoming mental health public forums and workshops and register online through the portal. The therapeutic games includes features such as immersing the child and adolescent in the role of an avatar, earning gold coins, having missions to accomplish to entice them to stay interested and engaged. "Saving Loumba" is literacy software designed to help ADHD child and adolescent with literacy difficulties learn ways to concentrate better and be less impulsive while engaged in reading and spelling activities. "Computer Assisted Strategies To Lessen Excessive Anxiety in Children (CASTLE-AC)" teaches child and adolescent skills in managing their anxiety through missions and quests to defeat anxiety monsters. Schools can subscribe to the games and can be trained on the use of the programme.

REACH often refers parents and school counsellors to ROC-N-ASH portal for more information. The ADHD module contains an ADHD screening tool that aids parents and school personnel in understanding whether child and adolescent's inattention and/or hyperactivity-impulsivity symptoms are severe and impairing enough to constitute a disorder. It also gives them a better understanding of the presentation of this disorder and trains school counsellors in picking up relevant ADHD symptoms. REACH uses the anxiety courseware to provide psycho-education to parents and CASTLE-AC forms part of our community interventions for child and adolescent with anxiety disorders.

ROC-N-ASH has received good feedback from school counsellors and parents who have used the portal. Many commented that the portal is well organised and easily understood by "non-experts" and found the detailed information and contents very useful and appealing. ROC-N-ASH is an easily accessible web portal that provides information on ADHD and anxiety disorders which helps enhance public's understanding of these common disorders. With improved knowledge, schools and parents are better able to identify symptoms of ADHD and anxiety in their children and students early in their presentations, learn how to help child and adolescent cope with their difficulties before it becomes worse, and provide necessary treatment promptly. With the game subscription, school counsellors are also equipped with an additional intervention tool that can aid in their counseling work with students. For mild cases, there would not be a need to be referred to CGC for treatment, minimising delayed treatment, saving time, transport costs and the need for parents to take leave. Therefore, REACH hopes that with the use of the web-portal, children facing difficulties with inattention/ impulsivity-hyperactivity and/or anxiety can conveniently benefit from early interventions in the community.

Case study

Rahim was a quiet and shy boy, and did not dare speak up in class. He was so shy, he did not know how to approach schoolmates who were playing games that he found interesting. All this was not of much concern until one day, Rahim was bullied on the school bus by a few older boys who were bigger in physique than he was. Rahim started becoming particularly fearful of his Mother Tongue class as he did not understand what the teacher was teaching and was often scolded when he gave the wrong answers in class. When Rahim was eleven years old, he became so afraid that he absolutely refused to go to school. He was then diagnosed to have anxiety disorder.

To help Rahim cope with his anxiety better, Rahim started therapy with a psychologist who used play with the anxiety management computer game, Roc-N-Ash, to support the learning of skills. In this role-playing game, Rahim assumed the avatar of a soldier who was to learn an array of anxiety coping skills based on CBT principles to fight the anxiety monsters in the game over eight therapy sessions. The skills taught included learning how to identify anxiety and anxious thoughts as well as coping with anxiety through relaxation strategies, coping statements and cognitive restructuring. Initially uninterested, Rahim became more motivated and engaged in therapy as he enjoyed playing the Roc-N-Ash computer game in the sessions.

Rahim's mother was also taught on how to help Rahim cope with his anxiety better using CBT and behavioural strategies during therapy sessions with the psychologist. In-between sessions, Rahim's mother was able to read materials available free on the ROC-N-ASH portal. As Rahim's father was not able to make it for most of the sessions due to work commitments, he was especially glad for this portal as he could access the free materials at any time of day to learn more about Rahim's difficulties and help to manage Rahim's anxiety.

Rahim's school was also able to access free materials written especially for school teachers on the same web portal. As a result, Rahim's school principal and class form teacher were more understanding of Rahim's condition and encouraged the school counsellor to help Rahim. Gradually, Rahim was able learn to work with his emotional issues and lower his anxiety and distress levels. He was, at last, able to return to school.

REACH website to support REACH partners and parents

REACH extended its services to the community by creating a website (http://www.reachforstudents.com), which was launched in 2010. Being online achieves a few purposes: publicity, providing information about REACH and its services, and serves as a tool to REACH's official partners (schools, VWO partners, General Practioner/GP partners).

As a service, REACH needs to find ways to increase awareness of the community about its availability. The website establishes an additional means for the public to understand and connect with the services that REACH provides to the community. For REACH partners, the website is a convenient way to introduce REACH services to families who will benefit from a referral to REACH. The website also provides a way for public to contact REACH to make enquiries or comments.

In addition, one of REACH's goals is to inform the public about what we do. It allows school counsellors, teachers, and various members of school administration to understand more about what we do beyond the courtesy visits that REACH makes to their school. For the parents, students, and concerned members of public, the website provides a safe way to find out more about REACH and how to get help for those who they think may need additional mental health support. REACH website also links the local community with useful websites that can provide more information about mental health conditions.

The website also serves as a one-stop resource portal for REACH's partners. REACH's partners can access quality material and resources that enhance their ability to support their care for the child and adolescent with mental health conditions whom they work with. They can also download the forms that they need for working with REACH, and are able to find useful rating scales and questionnaires that they can use in their own mental health care practice.

REACH is constantly working on improving its services to the child and adolescent. REACH website shares psychoeducational material for the general public to help them understand and recognise mental health conditions in children and adolescents, as well as learn about simple strategies that they can use to be of help. In the REACH website, detailed information about REACH and its services are available to help parents, schools, and child and adolescent to feel more comfortable knowing what to expect in a referral to REACH. Media presence is also celebrated on the website with postings of the latest news articles featuring REACH. The website is a way of reaching out those who may benefit from REACH's services to improve access and to support the mental health needs of Singapore's young.

Linking up with research programmes

Longitudinal Youth-at-Risk Study (LYRIKS)

Serious mental illness such as psychosis typically has its onset during the critical development period of adolescence and young adulthood. If untreated, it can lead to significant deterioration in the functioning of the affected individual. As with most illnesses, prevention, early detection and treatment will improve quality of life and chances of recovery. In 2008, the National Research Foundation of Singapore awarded funding to IMH to conduct a Flagship Translational and Clinical Research Programme in Neuroscience. This included the Longitudinal Youth At-Risk Study (LYRIKS — www.lyriks.com.sg), a community-based participatory research study that aims to identify key genetic, biological, cognitive, clinical, and social risk factors for serious mental illness. The findings from this study will enhance mental health professionals' knowledge of key risk factors associated with the development of serious mental illnesses, so that individuals who possess these risk factors can be identified early and receive appropriate preventive interventions.

LYRIKS involves the follow-up of a large group of youths with psychological and emotional difficulties over a period of two years. To be eligible for the study, participants have to be between 14–29 years old, completed at least Primary 6 education and are English-speaking. In addition, they must not have any head injury or neurological disorder, and are experiencing some psychological and emotional difficulties in the past one year. During this two-year period, comprehensive research assessments are completed at predetermined times. These research assessments consist of clinical and cognitive assessments, brain imaging, and genetic analyses of blood samples. Research participants who have been assessed to have developed any serious mental health problems during their participation in LYRIKS will be referred to the relevant clinical service for further help.

The LYRIKS screening tool, which helps professionals to identify youths with emotional difficulties and determine their eligibility to participate in the study, is used by REACH as part of its assessment of students with at-risk mental states. If a student is identified as a potential participant of LYRIKS, REACH will contact LYRIKS with the consent of the parents and assent of the youth to conduct a thorough screening interview in the community. If eligible, the student is encouraged to participate in LYRIKS. This screening tool is also made available to school counsellors, accompanied by a short instruction manual with guidelines on how to administer the screening tool. REACH recommends school counsellors to incorporate this screening tool into their routine assessment with students to help them get a rough understanding of the mental health of these students.

REACH helps to spread the word about LYRIKS in the community so that youths with emotional difficulties will come to learn about the study and consider contributing to the study as a research participant. With the use of the LYRIKS screening tool, school counsellors can have a better understanding of their students' mental health. In addition, through REACH's collaboration with LYRIKS, students with at-risk mental health can also be followed up accordingly.

Supplements and Social Skills Intervention Study (SASSI)

Conduct Disorder (CD) in children, characterised by a persistent pattern of antisocial behaviors, is a major predisposition to adult crime and violence. There is also substantial evidence for co-morbidity between CD and ADHD. Traditional treatment programmes for CD have focused on social and psychological processes, with variable degrees of success. More recently, an increasing body of neurobiological research has demonstrated a significant brain basis to antisocial behavior, both in children and adults.

Supplements And Social Skills Intervention (SASSI) Study is a research study under CGC investigating the use of nutritional and social skills intervention on child and adolescent with disruptive behavioural disorders. It is the first to test the efficacy of conjoint Omega-3/Social Skills treatment programme, and the first to identify possible mechanisms by which Omega-3 reduces antisocial behavior in child and adolescent in Singapore. SASSI was started in 2009, funded by the National Medical Research Council in Singapore and led by Dr Daniel Fung. The SASSI study has recruited 270 participants and has stopped recruitment since Aug 2012.

Children and youths who are between 9–16 years old with a minimum IQ of 70, diagnosed with Oppositional Defiant Disorder (ODD), CD and/or ADHD, are recruited in the study and randomly assigned to one of the four different treatment groups:

1. Omega 3 + Standard Parent Training
2. Omega 3 + Social Skills + Standard Parent Training
3. Placebo pill + Social Skills + Standard Parent Training
4. Placebo pill + Standard Parent Training

The children and their parents are required to attend a total of nine visits for this study which will last for one year.

Students who are assessed by REACH in schools and diagnosed with disruptive behavior disorders (ADHD, ODD, CD) will be referred to CGC for SASSI if parents are keen. These students will be seen by the REACH Medical Officer (MO) in CGC who will then inform SASSI clinicians to contact the parents to provide further details and get their consent to participate in the study.

REACH's collaboration with SASSI means that children with disruptive behaviors can be quickly linked up with the necessary programme designed to help them, without having to go through the long referral process to CGC. From REACH's experience, SASSI is a good alternative treatment programme for parents who are not keen to put their children on medication. Furthermore, in all treatment groups, parents can benefit from the standard parenting programme which teaches them skills and strategies in managing their children's disruptive behaviors. REACH also increases schools' awareness of this treatment programme so that school counsellors can refer children suitable for this programme through REACH. In this way, REACH bridges the information gap between community and clinic.

Drawings by students

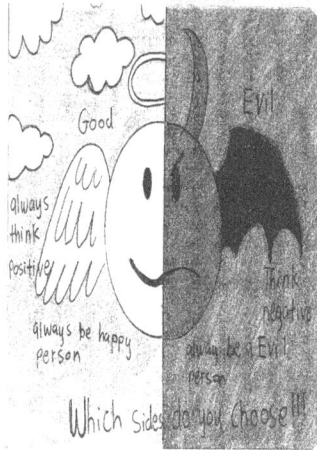

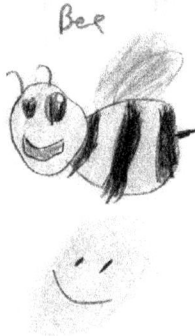

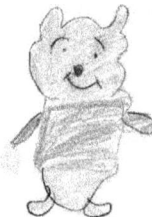

Resources

Drawings by students

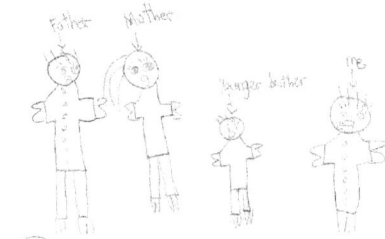

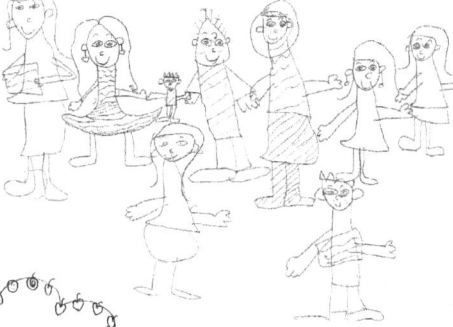

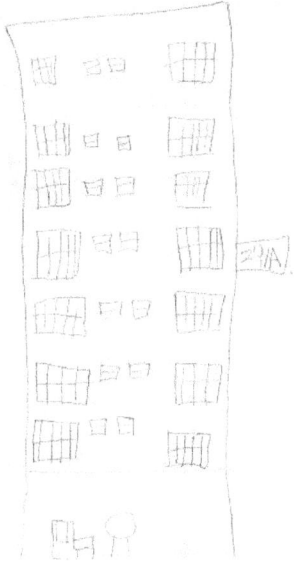

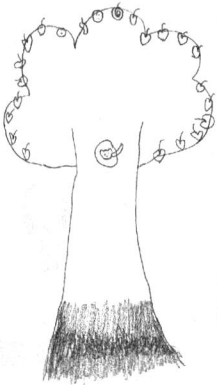

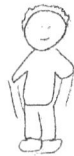

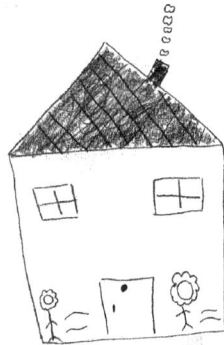

Chapter 7

Taking Stock and REACHing Beyond

Delphine Koh, Jillian Boon,
Daniel Fung, John Wong,
Chan Mei Chern, Cheak Ching Cheng and
Han Bing Ling

REACH Today

The REACH programme began as a vision of providing a mental health service for children, characterised by its accessibility and convenience within the natural setting of the child or adolescent. Starting with implementation in 12 pilot schools in the North Zone in 2007, the REACH programme was rolled out into the schools in the respective zones — South Zone in 2009, East Zone in 2010 and West Zone in 2011. To date, the REACH programme, comprising a team of more than 60 mental health professionals, is accessible to more than 350 schools in Singapore.

The development of REACH provides more than clinical services — it offers opportunities to build closer working relationships across sectors and agencies, and it is an enriching learning process for all who take part. Looking back over the past five years, the REACH programme has come a long way since it was first introduced to the school clusters in the North Zone. The journey thus far has raised some learning points that are significant for future directions and considerations.

Learning point 1: A stepped model of care is effective in improving mental health of children and adolescents in the community

Ensuring that the REACH programme is effective in meeting its objectives is an ongoing process. Various sources of data were captured to track the effectiveness of the REACH programme since its inception in 2007. Key Performance Indicators (KPIs), measuring both process and outcomes, were decided upon for each objective. These KPIs act as markers to monitor if goals were attained for each objective. The KPIs chosen were simple to monitor and reflected the intent of measurement.

Data collected indicated that the REACH programme had been successful in achieving its overarching goal of improving the emotional and social wellbeing of children and adolescents in Singapore. This was done through providing prompt delivery of services using a community-based approach. Over the last five years, over 1476 students suspected to have mental health issues were seen by REACH, and over half of these students were managed in the community. With the REACH programme, less than half of the referred students required a referral to a tertiary clinic specialising in child mental health. Figure 1 shows the number of helpline calls received, number of cases referred to REACH and number of cases referred to IMH and NUH from March 2007 to March 2012 across all four REACH teams.

In addition, the clinical effectiveness of the REACH programme was demonstrated through the improvements on ratings in clinical markers of mental health. Previously, small-scale research on clinical outcomes of youths referred through schools and managed by REACH had demonstrated the clinical effectiveness of the programme (Koh *et al.*, 2011; Sulaiman *et al.*, 2009). A more recent statistical analysis using pair-wise t-tests analyses on the pre-assessment and post-six months data from July 2007 to December 2011 also indicated positive improvements on the markers of mental health. More than half of referred youths from schools who went through the REACH

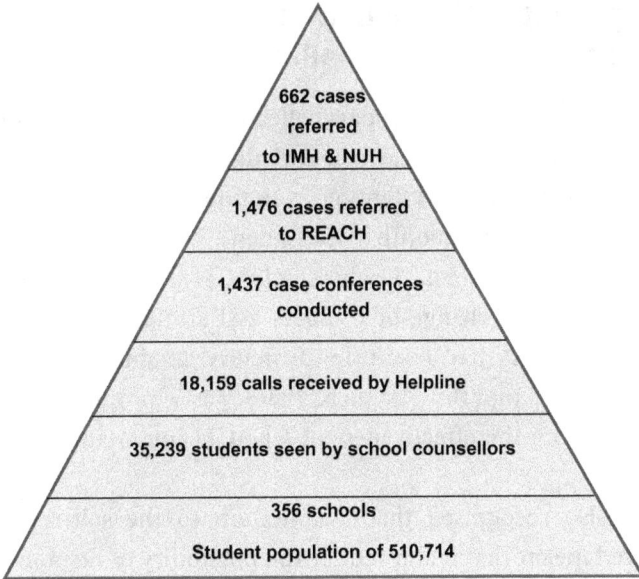

Figure 1   Stepped care model of primary mental health

programme showed improvement in their emotional and behavioural symptoms as indicated by the SDQ. Similar overall improvements in mental health as indicated on the CGI were noted six months after the first assessment by the REACH team. Likewise, all cases referred by VWO partners showed improvement in these same clinical indicators since the REACH VWO partnership started in Financial Year (FY) 2010.

With regard to the youths referred to REACH GP partners, over two-thirds of these referred students were rated by the GPs to have improved in their overall mental health. A majority of children and youths referred to GP partners every year were rated as having improved in their general functioning, with the exception of FY 2010, where only 25% showed improvement.

Ongoing data monitoring and research is being conducted by REACH to further examine the clinical effectiveness of the REACH programme.

Learning point 2: Evaluation of outcomes is necessary but can be challenging

Although it was recognised that data collection was essential in programme and outcome evaluation, it was acknowledged that various obstacles and limitations were brought to attention from time to time.

Collecting post-six months assessment evaluation measures from respective stakeholders (e.g., teachers, REACH partners) were at times a challenge. Inevitably, change of teachers and students leaving the school account for factors that result in difficulty attaining post evaluation measures after six months. As such, there was a proportion of students referred for whom the effectiveness of REACH intervention could not be ascertained.

It was also recognised that a limitation to the self-report surveys administered meant that it allowed for the possibility of response bias. The response bias of each rater (e.g., teachers and REACH partners) could affect the validity and generalisation of our outcome findings. As such, the ratings should be viewed with some caution.

Another limitation to consider was the lack of differentiation made into the specific diagnosis in relation to the improvements perceived by the school and REACH partners. The statistics provided a good general over-view of the improvements made by the students referred to REACH from various levels (primary, secondary and junior college). Although the improvements signify a good indication of attaining REACH's objectives, it would be helpful to understand the specific disorders that benefited most from REACH services. As such, future considerations can include the filtering of various disorders and the improvements measured.

Learning point 3: Planning for information management as an enabler is important

As data was captured to monitor the progress of REACH since 2007, a database using Microsoft Excel was initially created by REACH in-house within IMH for information management. However, as the REACH programme developed and expanded beyond IMH to include KKH and NUH, there was a need to develop a database that could be shared across various hospitals with the consent of parents. One consideration was to create a web-based database with internet connection for easy access by IMH, KKH and NUH in real time. This was challenging as it was necessary to safeguard the confidentiality of sensitive mental health information, and ensure that the web-based database was highly secured to meet the IT guidelines for management of patient information. Requirements on the database were complex. It would need to be user-friendly, provide capabilities to generate standard and customised statistical reports quickly, and allow easy retrieval of information such as the progress of student, the cases a staff member has handled, or the cases that need follow-up action. In addition, the database should be aligned with the existing workflow and processes of REACH. The information system would have to support the teams from each hospital to access student records under their care, and at the same time, enable designated administrators to have access to data from the four teams, and generate consolidated reports based on real time information.

A key challenge was in the identification of vendors with a proven track record in database development for the healthcare sector, while keeping costs manageable. There were limited vendors with healthcare experience then and they were usually big players in the market who charge at a premium. Through various sources and contacts, REACH was able to appoint a vendor who had a licensed software arrangement with an established Customer Relations Management (CRM) developer and also had experience working with healthcare institutions. The vendor was able to meet the complex needs of REACH and to come up with a database catered to our unique needs.

As the database contained information of students who may subsequently be referred to the hospital, the next challenge will be to create an interface to the hospital patient management systems maintained by IMH, KKH and NUH separately. This would be considered as the next phase of development for the database to integrate with the hospital appointment system (which is complex and designed differently for each hospital), while still keeping community records in the REACH database separate from the hospitals. All of this has to be done in a way that maintains privacy and confidentiality of information remained secure at all times.

Learning point 4: Training and capacity building is an effective lever to improve mental healthcare

A holistic approach to empowering partners in the community was taken when providing support and trainings to partners in the community (i.e., school counsellors, VWOs and GP partners). Trainings do not merely encompass didactic style lectures but also include practice of skills learnt and case consultations. As capacity building is important to ensure that mental health knowledge is cascaded from REACH to the various community partners, it was a deliberate cost strategy to offer trainings to REACH partners (i.e., school counsellors, VWOs and GPs partners) at no cost to encourage greater participation.

REACH team members conduct regular workshops covering topics ranging from clinical interviewing to the various childhood mental health disorders. In addition, training sessions usually reserved for clinical staff of hospitals were often extended to REACH partners as well. For instance, under the MOH Health Manpower Development Plan, internationally renowned professionals in their fields of expertise were invited from time to time to conduct intensive training for a week to hospital staff. It is now the practice that a number of these training sessions are open to REACH community partners, to ensure that they are kept updated on international best practices as well. Similarly, community partners were strongly encouraged to attend the monthly interagency case conference held at the Child Guidance Clinic, Health Promotion Board. The monthly interagency case conference is an anonymised case presentation which highlights particular cases with greater complexities. Participation and attendance in these case conferences allow partners to partake in a multidisciplinary exchange of ideas. To ensure that REACH trainings were relevant to the work done by community partners, school counsellors and VWO partners were asked after every training session they attended if they had found the training to be satisfactory and effective. Consistently, more than 90% of school counsellors and VWO staff who attended REACH trainings felt that the trainings had been effective in providing them necessary skills and were satisfied with the trainings provided.

Another avenue of support for school counsellors and VWO partners is the case conferences on management planning for children and adolescents referred to REACH. These case conferences are now the routine after the assessment of each child, to ensure that the school counsellors or VWO partner is involved and supported in the future management of the child.

Learning point 5: A network of community partners for REACH can be built upon a foundation of roll-out in mainstream schools

The REACH teams began with a focus on providing community mental health services to mainstream schools and building up the capabilities of school counsellors. Working with the mainstream schools allowed REACH to develop along the well-established infrastructure of MOE. REACH could leverage on school-based communication channels and regular meetings to implement processes and refine them based on feedback collated from the schools. For example, the REACH team designed templates for mainstream schools to guide them in giving relevant information when making referrals. This template went through multiple revisions to reach a state that ensures that succinct yet comprehensive information is provided by the school counsellors, so as to facilitate effective triage by the REACH team. The rigour of this earlier revision benefited the implementation of the referral and triage process with the VWO partners and SPED schools. The triage template was readily customised to meet the needs of the VWOs and SPED schools.

As another example, the need for school visits to engage leaders of mainstream schools proved to be instrumental in the subsequent successful roll out to VWOs and SPED schools. Support from the leaders of these agencies/ schools enabled smooth adoption of REACH referral processes by other personnel e.g. teachers who were not directly trained by REACH, and more timely submission of documentation required by REACH.

Similarly, training programmes were first developed for school counsellors during the implementation with schools in the North and South zones, and later fine-tuned for subsequent implementations with schools in the remaining zones, VWOs and SPED schools. The set of training materials from the first phase of training provided a base which could be quickly customised for the varied needs of partners who came on board the REACH network later. Further, assessment and intervention of referrals by mainstream schools provided avenues for live observation by participants of later training programmes. Among the training programme for the VWOs, field observation was an important component. Social workers and pro-gramme managers from VWOs obtained direct exposure to mental health assessment with the provision of opportunities to shadow REACH team members to school.

The next steps

Ongoing enrichment of service offerings and leveraging on new resources

REACHing out to the community is a continuous effort. Developing and strengthening new and existing partnerships must continue. Similarly, coming up with innovative and community-based training, assessments and interventions would be an ongoing mission of REACH. One such effort in community-based training was the development of group-based training in parenting for children with specific diagnoses.

To meet the needs of children and adolescents ranging from mild to severe forms of mental illnesses, several external agencies, services and programmes have surfaced. Inevitably, some of these programmes offered have an overlap in the services provided. For instance, the establishment of the National Addictions Service (NAMS) adolescent clinic looks into assessing youths with dependence-related issues. Concurrently, REACH has had progressive referrals of students with mental health issues with underlying addiction problems (e.g. computer addiction). Here, the overlap of services comes where assessment or intervention can be provided within the community as well as in-house in a clinic which specialises in addic-tions. As such, greater efforts to communicate and collaborate will be necessary to enable that the students referred get the most appropriate help.

To eradicate institutional problems of overlap in service provision and the lack of communication, transparency of care where information about services provided should be readily available to consumers (i.e. teachers, parents, and

REACH partners) and allied health professionals. This way, informed decisions can be made as to what is expected in terms of the specialisation of the various departments and external agencies where appropriate partnerships and collaborations can be made in view of the multi-faceted nature of mental illnesses.

Our ever-evolving society has brought on new challenges with the rise of new conditions. For instance, internet and gaming addictions at this point is a growing problem but lacks evidence-based treatment processes that have been validated in Asian populations. Thus, there is a growing need to expand our services to accommodate these new conditions through integration and collaboration of services.

According to Chan (2010), statistics highlighted that 'one in ten will suffer from mental illness'. Particularly, several adult mental health issues have an early onset, starting from a young age. Therefore, an increase in internal awareness within the institutional departments as well as external agencies is necessary to increase greater understanding of the progression of mental illnesses. To reiterate, this would be best done through collaboration and partnership between existing programmes.

To strengthen the partnership network, collaboration with existing programmes that target specific youth population is important. One of such collaboration leverages on the NAMS adolescent clinic named RELIVE, which attends to adolescents age between 13 to 19, who need help with behavioural (e.g., computer and gambling) and also substance addictions (e.g., alcohol and drugs). Many youths and their parents may not be keen to go to NAMS for treatment due to stigma. NAMS collaborates with REACH to disseminate information to the schools via full-time school counsellors. This aims to enhance knowledge on how to identify adolescents who are at risk of addictions, encourage adolescents at risk of addictions to seek treatment, and empower desperate parents to seek help. Moving on, REACH hopes to facilitate the support for adolescents between clinic and the community. More ways could be explored to work closely with NAMS to support an adolescent's reintegration back to school and to provide support for adolescents with addiction problems in the community. REACH will also continue building networks with VWOs and other community partners to support these adolescents and their family at a community level.

REACHing beyond low-hanging fruits

The school-based community teams are now well-accepted members of the educational and counselling community. However, the linkages between GP partners and the social agencies would need more work. One of the difficulties lies in the stigma of mental health which prevents many partners from engaging REACH services. As a result, a more health-based system of engagement may be necessary. For younger children, a developmental framework may be the best opportunity for this to work. Using the developmental screening programme that is currently imple-mented at the preschool age group, and incorporating mental health screening within such a framework may be the way to accomplish such an engagement.

Another possible method of engagement may be to use a family-based approach in providing care. Adults who seek medical services could be screened on their psychosocial needs and relevant linkages with social agen-cies trained to identify mental health disorders could be made. Such an intervention would need cross-trained social workers and family physi-cians. A Graduate Diploma in Mental Health was launched in 2010 and is now into its third run. With an increasing pool of such cross trained profes-sionals, the primary mental health needs of children and their families could be readily met.

The planning for a preschool programme similar to REACH but work-ing with preschools and childcare centres throughout Singapore has begun. More than 1000 such facilities exist and would represent a logistical chal-lenge to reach out to all of them.

The business of public healthcare

The key to sustaining a successful idea that has been operationalised is to make sure that it stays in place even after the initial pilot funding is complete. In order to sustain the programme, regular budget funding from the government is necessary. In Singapore, a co-payment approach has been adopted in all public areas including education and health.

Greater integration of services in child developmental services

The plan for the future is to re-engineer the role of hospital services and the CGC to become focal points of a regional mental healthcare system for children and adolescents. The four zones of Singapore will be supported by IMH, KKH and NUH, giving a vertically integrated network for delivering services, as shown in Figure 2. Connecting with psychiatric services of other general public hospitals in different geographical locations will also facilitate accessibility of secondary mental health care and convenience for students and their families. As an example, REACH North has recently formalised a collaboration with Khoo Teck Puat Hospital located in the Northern part of Singapore. This collaboration would mean that suitable students who live in the northern region can be referred for subsidised psychiatric services after a mental health assessment has been conducted by REACH. The integration aims to achieve greater effectiveness in the allocation of scarce resources. More importantly, it would establish a comprehensive and holistic child and adolescent mental health delivery system that supports the child and his family through various stages of the child and the family's development.

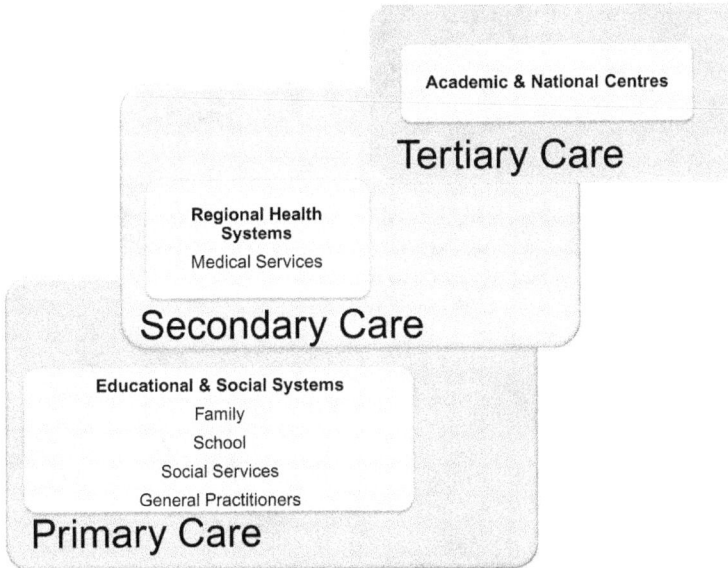

Academic & National Centres

Tertiary Care

Regional Health Systems

Medical Services

Secondary Care

Educational & Social Systems

Family

School

Social Services

General Practitioners

Primary Care

Figure 2.   Vision toward more integrated child developmental services

Faces of REACH

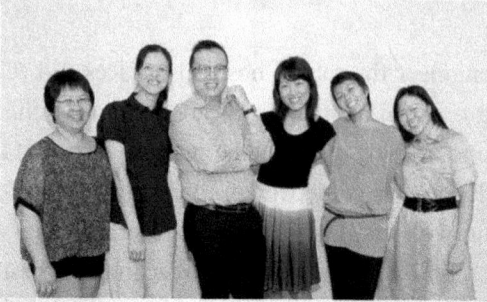

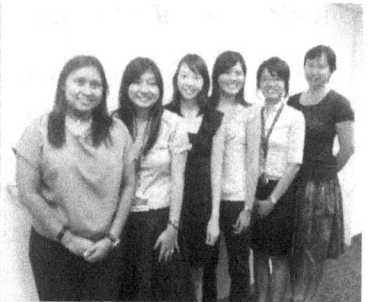

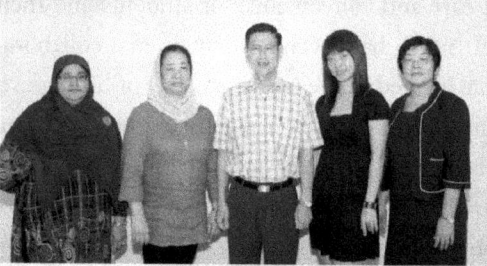

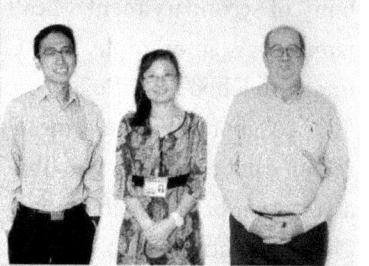

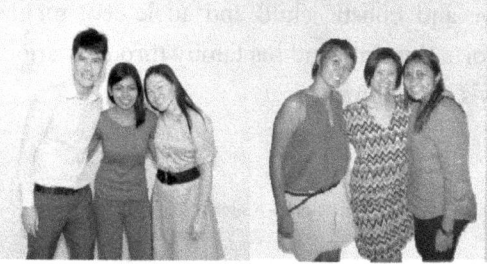

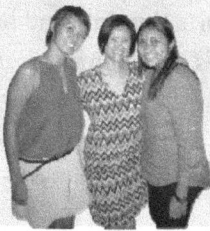

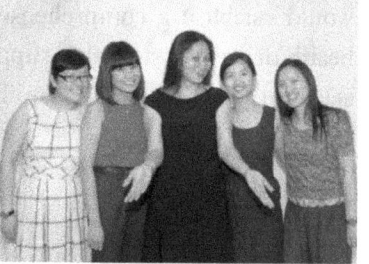

Abbreviations for Key Institutions and Organisations

APCATS	*Aged Psychiatry Community Assessment and Treatment Service (IMH)*
ARC	*Autism Resource Centre*
CGC	*Child Guidance Clinic (IMH)*
CMHT	*Community Mental Health Team (IMH)*
FSC	*Family Service Centre*
GB	*Guidance Branch (MOE)*
HPB	*Health Promotion Board*
IMH	*Institute of Mental Health*
KKH	*KK Women's and Children's Hospital*
KTPH	*Khoo Teck Puat Hospital*
MCYS*	*Ministry of Community, Youth Development, and Sports*
MINDS	*Movement for the Intellectually Disabled of Singapore*
MOE	*Ministry of Education*
MOH	*Ministry of Health*
NCSS	*National Council of Social Services*
NUH	*National University Hospital*
PSB	*Psychological Services Branch (MOE)*
REACH	*Response, Early intervention, and Assessment in Community mental Health*
SPED	*Special Education (School)*
WHO	*World Health Organisation*
VWO	*Voluntary Welfare Organisation*

*Note: As of 1 November 2012, MCYS will be renamed the Ministry of Social and Family Development (MSF).

Glossary of Mental Disorders in REACH Chronicles

Anxiety/Anxiety disorders	*Anxiety is a feeling of worry, unease, and tension about possible danger. Anxiety disorders are defined by excessive or prolonged anxiety to any perceived threats. Types of anxiety disorders include Separation Anxiety Disorder (See Separation Anxiety Disorder), Social Phobia (See Social Phobia), and others.*
Attention Deficit Hyperactivity Disorder (ADHD)	*A neurobehavioural disorder characterised by persistent difficulties in sustaining attention and/or excessive motor activity and impulsive behaviours across different settings.*
Autism Spectrum Disorders	*A group of disorders characterised by difficulties in verbal and non-verbal communication and social interaction skills, as well as restricted and repetitive interests and activities. Also known as Pervasive Developmental Disorder and includes Autistic Disorder and Asperger's Disorders.*
Conduct Disorder (CD)	*A disorder where the child or young person consistently behaves in a manner that is against societal norms and rules. This includes behaviours such as aggression towards other people and/or animals, destroying property, stealing and lying, truancy, and running away from home.*

Depression	*While depression can be used to describe a mood state of feeling depressed or very sad, it is clinically used to describe a disorder characterised by a prolonged state of depressed or irritable mood, loss of interest or pleasure, changes in appetite or sleep, feelings of worthlessness and guilt, low energy, and poor concentration. Depression is a type of Mood Disorder.*
Dyslexia	*A type of learning disorder, also known as Reading Disorder, where the child's reading ability is significantly poorer than that expected based on his or her age, intelligence, and education.*
Eating Disorders	*A group of disorders characterised by disturbed eating behaviours and distorted body image. Anorexia Nervosa involves excessive dieting or exercising despite a low body weight whereas Bulimia Nervosa involves binge eating followed by various methods to overcompensate previous food intake such as self-induced vomiting.*
Learning disorders/ learning difficulty	*A group of disorders where the child's reading, mathematical, or writing ability is significantly poorer than that expected based on his or her age, intelligence, or education.*
Mental health	*"A state of well-being in which every individual realizes his or her own potential, can cope with the normal stresses of life, can work productively and fruitfully, and is able to make a contribution to her or his community"* *(WHO, 2007).*

Mental disorders	*A mental disorder is "a clinically significant behavioural or psychological syndrome or pattern that occurs in an individual and that is associated with present distress or disability or with a significantly increased risk of suffering death, pain, disability, or an important loss of freedom. This syndrome or pattern must not be merely an expectable and culturally sanctioned response to a particular event. Whatever its original cause, it must be considered as a manifestation of a behavioural, psychological, or biological dysfunction in the individual." (APA, 2000, p. xxxi).*
	Mental disorders can only be diagnosed by trained mental health professionals according to diagnostic criteria set out in the current versions of either the Diagnostic and Statistical Manual of Mental Disorders — Fourth Edition Text Revision (DSM-IV TR) (APA, 2000) or the International Statistical Classification of Diseases and Related Health Problems Tenth Revision (ICD — 10) (WHO, 2010).
Mood disorders	*A group of disorders where the predominant disturbances are in how the child or young person is feeling. See Depression.*
Oppositional Defiant Disorder (ODD)	*A disorder where the child or young person consistently antagonizes, defies, and disobeys authority figures such as parents and teachers.*
Psychosis/ Psychotic Disorders	*Psychosis or psychotic symptoms refer to distortions in thought content (delusions) or in perception (hallucinations). Delusions include false beliefs about what is going on and who one is, and hallucinations include having sensory perceptions such as hearing and seeing things that are not actually there. Psychotic Disorders refer to a group of disorders characterised by psychosis or psychotic symptoms.*

Pervasive Developmental Disorders	*See Autism Spectrum Disorders.*
Separation Anxiety Disorder (SAD)	*An anxiety disorder where the child experiences a lot of anxiety when he or she experiences or anticipates temporary separation from home or from those to whom he or she is attached to (usually parents).*
Selective Mutism	*A disorder characterised by a lack of speech in selected social settings despite fluent speech in others.*
Social Phobia	*An anxiety disorder characterised by persistent and excessive worries about being evaluated negatively by others in social settings or when the child or young person has to perform in front of others. Also known as Social Anxiety Disorder.*

Appendix A
Role descriptions of REACH team members

The REACH Multidisciplinary Team — Description of the scope and focus of each role in the REACH team

Statement of Purpose (for psychologist, medical social worker, community psychiatric nurse (children and adolescents) and occupational therapist):

1. to improve the mental health of children and adolescents in schools by providing early intervention and assessment to students
2. to equip school counsellors with skills to manage students with mental health conditions at school, and
3. to develop a mental health network for children and adolescents in the community involving:

   a. GPs
   b. school counsellors
   c. VWOs and SPED Schools.

Psychologist

(A) Specific (80%)

Clinical role

1. triage new cases and provide advice to school counsellors, identified staff in the SPED schools and VWO partners on helpline
2. provide input and expertise during multidisciplinary team discussion for new cases and existing cases that present with problems
3. conduct initial clinical assessment and clerking
4. conduct cognitive assessment
5. provide support, training and guidance in implementation of therapeutic interventions to school counsellors through telephone advice/consultation, case conferences talks or workshops
6. provide individual psychological therapy for clinical/psychiatric disorders
7. provide group therapy

Case management role

1. formulate and develop care management plans for referred students in collaboration with school counsellors and other community partners
2. support clinicians in right-siting suitable students to GPs for follow up
3. coordinate all aspects of transfer of care, from referral to the first GP clinical visit and to monitor the right-sited student's attendance
4. collaborate with GPs to evaluate the student's adherence to the treatment, and support GP in evaluating programme outcomes

Liaison role

1. initiate appropriate referral and liaison with other healthcare professionals and agencies
2. establish a network of resources and information for dissemination to the referred student/caregiver and school counsellor

(B) General (20%)

1. to serve on specific task force(s) designated by the hospital
2. to conduct research independently and/or in collaboration with fellow professionals
3. to carry out projects and duties assigned by REACH Team Leader, Deputy Head or Head of Department of Psychology.

Medical Social Worker

(A) Specific (80%)

Clinical role

1. triage new cases and provide advice to school counsellors, identified staff in the SPED schools and VWO partners on helpline
2. provide input and expertise during multidisciplinary team discussion for new cases and existing cases that present with problems
3. conduct bio-psychosocial assessment to determine selected students' current mental state
4. provide support, training and guidance in implementation of therapeutic interventions to school counsellors through telephone advice/consultation, case conferences talks or workshops
5. provide individual and family therapy for clinical/psychiatric disorders
6. provide group therapy

Case management role

1. formulate and develop care management plans for referred students in collaboration with school counsellors and other community partners
2. support clinicians in right-siting suitable students to GPs for follow up
3. coordinate all aspects of transfer of care, from referral to the first GP clinical visit and to monitor the right-sited student's attendance
4. collaborate with GPs to evaluate the student's adherence to the treatment, and support GP in evaluating programme outcomes

Liaison role

1. initiate appropriate referral and liaison with other healthcare professionals and agencies
2. establish a network of resources and information for dissemination to the referred student/caregiver and school counsellor

(B) General (20%)

1. to serve on specific task force(s) designated by the hospital
2. to conduct research independently and/or in collaboration with fellow professionals
3. to carry out projects and duties assigned by REACH Team Leader, Deputy Head or Head of Department of Medical Social Work.

Community Psychiatric Nurse (Children and Adolescents)

(A) Specific (80%)

Clinical role

1. triage new cases and provide advice to school counsellors, identified staff in the SPED schools and VWO partners on helpline
2. conduct bio-psychosocial assessment to determine selected students' current mental state
3. provide psychological support and intervention to the referred students and caregivers
4. monitor and evaluate referred student's progress and revise treatment/care plan as needed
5. provide support, training and guidance in implementation of therapeutic interventions to school counsellors through telephone advice/consultation, case conferences talks or workshops

Case management role

1. formulate and develop care management plans for referred students in collaboration with school counsellors and other community partners

2. support clinicians in right-siting suitable students to GPs for follow up
3. coordinate all aspects of transfer of care, from referral to the first GP clinical visit and to monitor the right-sited student's attendance
4. collaborate with GPs to evaluate the student's adherence to the treatment, and support GP in evaluating programme outcomes

Liaison role

1. initiate appropriate referral and liaison with other healthcare professionals and agencies
2. establish a network of resources and information for dissemination to the referred student/caregiver and school counsellor

(B) Non-specific (20%)

Quality Management

1. assist in formulation and revision of guidelines, standards and procedures
2. participate in quality improvement projects

General

1. maintain a database of students referred or managed by the multidisciplinary team
2. function as a clinical resource to all members of the team
3. perform any other assigned duty by Assistant Director of Nursing.

Occupational Therapist

(A) Specific (80%)

Clinical role

1. triage new cases and provide advice to school counsellors, identified staff in the SPED schools and VWO partners on helpline
2. provide input and expertise during multidisciplinary team discussion for new cases and existing cases that present with problems

3. provide initial clinical assessment and clerking
4. provide appropriate occupational therapy assessments (e.g. handwriting, functional sensory, visual perception, fine motor/motor, environmental assessments)
5. provide support, training and guidance in implementation of therapeutic interventions to school counsellors through telephone advice/consultation, case conferences talks or workshops
6. provide individual occupational therapy interventions for students referred
7. provide group therapy

Case management role

1. formulate and develop care management plans for referred students in collaboration with school counsellors and other community partners
2. support clinicians in right-siting suitable students to GPs for follow up
3. coordinate all aspects of transfer of care, from referral to the first GP clinical visit and to monitor the right-sited student's attendance
4. collaborate with GPs to evaluate the student's adherence to the treatment, and support GP in evaluating programme outcomes

Liaison role

1. initiate appropriate referral and liaison with other healthcare professionals and agencies
2. establish a network of resources and information for dissemination to the referred student/caregiver and school counsellor

(B) General (20%)

1. to serve on specific task force(s) designated by the hospital
2. to conduct research independently and/or in collaboration with fellow professionals
3. to carry out projects and duties assigned by REACH Team Leader, Deputy Head or Head of Department of Occupational Therapy.

Medical Officer

Statement of Purpose: to provide treatment to child and adolescent psychiatric patients in the community. The medical officer is a trainee/resident in psychiatry.

Major duties and responsibilities
1. provide medical advice to the members of the REACH team at team meetings and at teaching sessions
2. provide medical support to members of the REACH team via triage of new cases on site (school or home visits)
3. clerking new cases referred by REACH Team to the outpatient clinic and reply to referring school counsellor/SPED/VWO partner on diagnosis, management
4. follow up of cases referred by REACH team with referring school counsellor/SPED/VWO partner
5. discuss cases seen in the clinic with Consultant of the REACH team

Project Director

Major duties and responsibilities

1. identify, develop and implement the health services and manpower development specific to the project
2. develop an implementation plan and time schedule
3. establish desired outcomes and key performance indicators with the Ministry of Health, and submit progress reports on stipulated frequency and milestones
4. submit financial budget projection in consultation with Director of Finance, and work in conjunction on financial management of the project
5. update Ministry of Health on changes to the financial requirement or outcome indicators to the project
6. provide information and assistance to Ministry of Health in its evaluation of the project
7. in the event that the project director leaves employment, to ensure a smooth handover to the appointed successor.

Director/Deputy Director/Assistant Director (Patient Operations)

Statement of purpose: to function as a key resource person, working in close collaboration with members of the multidisciplinary team, to develop and implement appropriate operational and administrative procedures and strategies to support clinical service delivery and quality initiatives in the assigned patient operations area (Aligned with clinical department), in line with the IMH vision and mission and MOH's long term strategic direction.

(A) Specific

1. provide leadership, set overall direction and oversee operations and administrative functions for the department
2. set standards for operations within the clinical department
3. plan, implement and administer programmes and services in the department
4. work in conjunction with Nursing and Ambulatory Services to determine staffing requirements, and where needed, recruit, train or oversee the relevant personnel processes
5. review and analyse facility activities and data to aid planning and management and to improve service utilisation
6. oversee the department's budget plans, manage funds utilisation and other performance data, and to ensure compliance with hospital and stakeholders' financial policies
7. establish and implement policies, goals, objectives and procedures in operations and administrative areas, and to conduct periodic reviews to improve service delivery and quality
8. work and coordinate closely with stakeholders, management members and clinicians in the department to deliver shared goals and overall strategic objectives

(B) General

1. cultivate a culture of learning by providing learning and development opportunities for staff
2. supervise and schedule work of staff, and promote harmonious working relationships to ensure effective performance and optimal productivity
3. undertake special projects or duties as assigned by Chief Operating Officer or Department Head

Manager/Assistant Manager/Senior Executive

Statement of purpose: to support the development and implementation of operational and administrative procedures and strategies that support clinical service delivery and quality initiatives.

(A) Specific

1. support the operational and administrative functions of the Department of Child and Adolescent Psychiatry (DCAP)
2. support the conceptualisation of business plan for new clinical programme
3. formulate, implement and review new and existing policies and processes to improve the efficiency of the department in its service quality and resource utilisation
4. assist in the development, monitoring, evaluation and maintenance of systems required to support operations
5. collaborate with relevant stakeholders to support the delivery of the clinic la programme and quality initiatives
6. work and coordinate closely with all key management members and clinicians in the department to deliver shared goals and overall strategic objectives

(B) General

1. perform any other duties as assigned within Department of Patient Operations and the DCAP.

Administrative Assistant

Statement of purpose: to provide administrative support to the REACH Team.

(A) Specific — Administrative (80%)

Coordination role

1. provide administrative functions including, but not limited to, writing minutes, printing and preparing training/resource materials
2. provide logistical functions including, but not limited to, sourcing for quotations, raising purchase requests, room booking and arrangement for refreshments
3. liaison with internal and external stakeholders for meetings, school/home visits
4. keep track and oversee maintenance of assets, equipment and inventories
5. record and update staff movement.

Supporting role

1. update statistical/data for tracking purposes
2. update patient records in the appointment systems required by REACH assessments/interventions
3. support clinicians in their administrative role e.g. tracing patient records, filing, serving reminders to patients for visits/payments, liaising with GPs
4. assist in managing the helpline when needed

(B) General (20%)

1. Others: any other administrative duties as assigned by supervisors in REACH team and in Department of Corporate Development.

Appendix B
List of Special Education Schools in Singapore

List of SPED Schools in Singapore

School	Address	Contact Information	Disability Groups	Age Group
AWWA School	11 Lorong Napiri Singapore 547532	Tel: (65) 6511 5280 Fax: (65) 6511 5281 awwaschool@awwa.org.sg	Multiple Disabilities; Autism	6–18 years old
Canossian School	No.1 Sallim Road Singapore 387621	Tel: (65) 6749 8971 Fax: (65) 6749 8976 admin@canossian.edu.sg	Hearing Impairment; Autism	6–18 years old
Chaoyang School	18 Ang Mo Kio Ave 9 Singapore 569767	Tel: (65) 6456 6922 Fax: (65) 6456 2030 cys@apsn.org.sg	Mild Intellectual Disability; Mild Autism	6–12 years old
Delta Senior School	20 Delta Avenue Singapore 169832	Tel: (65) 6276 3818 Fax: (65) 6276 5608 dss@apsn.org.sg	Intellectual Disability	17–18/ 21 years old
Eden School	101 Bukit Batok West Avenue 3 Singapore 659168	Tel: (65) 6265 7400 Fax: (65) 6265 9400 enquiry@edenschool.edu.sg	Autism	6–18 years old
Fernvale Gardens School	7 Fernvale Road Singapore 797635	Tel: (65) 6481 6697 Fax: (65) 6483 2631 fgs@minds.org.sg	Moderate Intellectual Disability; Moderate Autism	6–18 years old
Grace Orchard School	6A Jurong West St 52 Singapore 649297	Tel: (65) 6561 9128 Fax: (65) 6561 4133 info@go.edu.sg	Mild Intellectual Disability; Mild Autism	6–18 years old
Katong School	900 New Upper Changi Road Singapore 467354	Tel: (65) 6445 8027 Fax: (65) 6445 6313 ks@apsn.org.sg	Mild Intellectual Disability; Mild Autism	6–18 years old

(Continued)

List of SPED Schools in Singapore (*Continued*)

School	Address	Contact Information	Disability Groups	Age Group
Lee Kong Chian Gardens School	802 Margaret Drive Singapore 149311	Tel: (65) 6473 8332 Fax: (65) 6473 4776 lgs@minds.org.sg	Moderate Intellectual Disability; Moderate Autism	6–18 years old
Metta School	30 Simei St 1 Singapore 529949	Tel: (65) 6788 5800 Fax: (65) 6788 5507 enquiry@mettaschool.edu.sg	Mild Intellectual Disability; Mild Autism	6–18/ 21 years old
Pathlight School	5 Ang Mo Kio Ave 10 Singapore 569739	Tel: (65) 6459 9951 Fax: (65) 6459 3397 queries@pathlight.org.sg	Autism	6–18/ 21 years old
Rainbow Centre — Margaret Drive School	501 Margaret Drive Singapore 149306	Tel: (65) 6472 7077 Fax: (65) 6475 9739 mdss@rainbowcentre.org.sg	Multiple Disabilities; Autism	6–18 years old
Rainbow Centre — Yishun Park School	15 Yishun Street 61 Singapore 768548	Tel: (65) 6482 2592 Fax: (65) 6482 2593 rcbs@rainbowcentre.org.sg	Multiple Disabilities; Autism	6–18 years old
Singapore School for the Deaf	227 Mountbatten Road Singapore 397998	Tel: (65) 6345 6765 Fax: (65) 6345 9095 admin@ssd.edu.sg	Hearing Impairment	6–18 years old
Lighthouse School	51 Toa Payoh Rise Singapore 298106	Tel: (65) 6250 3755 Fax: (65) 6250 5348 lighthouse@lighthouse.edu.sg	Visual Impairment; Autism; Hearing Impairment	6–18 years old
Spastic Children's Association School	65 Pasir Ris Drive 1 Singapore 519529	Tel: (65) 6585 5639 Fax: (65) 6585 5635 spastic@pacific.net.sg	Physical Disability	6–18 years old
St Andrew's Autism School	1 Elliott Road Singapore 458686	Tel: (65) 6517 3800 Fax: (65) 6517 3801	Autism	6–18 years old
Tanglin School	143 Alexandra Road Singapore 159924	Tel: (65) 6475 1511 Fax: (65) 6472 0408 ts@apsn.org.sg	Mild Intellectual Disability, Mild Autism	13–18 years old
Towner Gardens School	1B Lengkong Lima Singapore 417557	Tel: (65) 6446 2612 Fax: (65) 6243 7498 tgs@minds.org.sg	Moderate Intellectual Disability; Moderate Autism	6–18 years old
Woodlands Gardens School	30 Woodlands Ring Road #01–01 Singapore 737883	Tel: (65) 6468 0566 Fax: (65) 6468 2142 wgs@minds.org.sg	Modearate Intellectual Disability; Moderate Autism	6–18 years old

Reference: Ministry of Education. (2010). List of Special Education Schools. In *Special Education*. Retrieved 30 November 2011 from http://www.moe.gov.sg/education/special-education/schoollist

Appendix C: List of REACH — VWO partners

VWO	Address	Services
MCYC Community Services Society	Blk 106 Bukit Batok Central #01-217, Singapore 650106	Children — Psychological Services — Learning Centre Youth — School-Based Services — Tuition Befriending — Youth Centre (YouthCan@mcyc) Parents — Parenting and Family Programmes — Community Events — Counselling Centre (EPYC@mcyc) URL: http://www.mcyc.sg/
Singapore Children's Society	Blk 107 Yishun Ring Rd, #01-233, Singapore 760107	Children Service Centre Tel: 6448 6658 Family Service Centre (Yishun) Tel: 6753 7331 Research and Outreach Centre Tel: 6358 0911 Round Box Tel: 6259 3735 Student Care Centre (Henderson) Tel: 6278 7856 Student Service Hub (Bukit Merah) Tel: 6276 5077

(Continued)

(Continued)

VWO	Address	Services
		Sunbeam Place Tel: 6462 3477 Youth Centre (Jurong) Tel: 6566 6989 Youth Service Centre (Toa Payoh) Tel: 6253 1124 Children's Medical Fund Helpdesk Tel: 6753 1083 Tinkle Friend Helpline Tel: 1800 2744 788 URL: http://www.childrensociety.org.sg/
Students Care Service (Hougang)	Blk 463 Hougang Ave 10 #01-964, Singapore 530463	Social Work Services — Casework and Counselling — Children, Preteens and Youth Programmes — Mentoring Programme — Guidance Programme — School-based Social Work Educational Psychology Services — Consultation and Diagnostic Assessment — Intervention Programmes — Developmental Programmes — Consultation and Workshops for Parents and Professionals Training and Consultancy Research and Publication URL: http://www.students.org.sg/
Students Care Service (Clementi)	Blk 437 Clementi Ave 3 #01-98, Singapore 120437	
Beyond Social Services	26 Jalan Klinik #01-42/52 Singapore, 160026	Juvenile Justice Family Services Supporting families with children and youth in conflict with the law and school URL: http://www.beyond.org.sg/
Persatuan Persuratan Pemuda Pemudi (4PM) Malay Youth Literary Association	Blk 606 Bedok Reservoir Road #01-716, Singapore 470606	Casework and Counselling Mentoring Enhanced Step Up URL: http://www.4pm.org.sg Email: secretariat@4pm.org.sg 4PM Education centre

(Continued)

(Continued)

VWO	Address	Services
Fei Yue Community Services	Multiple locations, Refer to:- http://www.fycs.org/index.cfm?GPID=36	Family Service Center Community Services Adoption Services Early Intervention Programmes (Infants and Children) Resource Speaker Family Life Education Services for Inmates and Their Families Youth Programmes Project 180 (Youth Services) Training

The above services are not exhaustive. Please visit the individual centres' websites for updated information.

References

Introduction

American Psychiatric Association (2000). *Diagnostic and statistical manual of mental disorders* (4th ed, text rev.). Washington, DC: Author.

Ang, R. P., & Fung, D. S. S. (2006). *Seeing Red: Help your child deal with anger at home and in public.* Singapore: SNP International.

Barkmann, C., & Schulte-Markwort, M. (2005). Emotional and behavioral problems of children and adolescents in Germany. *Social psychiatry and psychiatric epidemiology, 40*(5), 357–366.

Burns, T. (2004). Community mental health teams. *Psychiatry, 3*(9), 11–14.

Cai, Y. M. (1998). Adolescent Suicide. *The Singapore Family Physician, 24*(2).

Cai, Y. M., & Fung, D. S. S. (1998). *Help your child to cope: understanding childhood stress.* Singapore: Times Books International.

Christiana, J., Gilman, S., Guardino, M., Mickelson, K., Morselli, P., Olfson, M., & Kessler, A. C. (2000). Duration between onset and time of obtaining initial treatment among people with anxiety and mood disorders: an international survey of members of mental health patient advocate groups. *Psychological Medicine, 30*(3), 693–703.

Chua, H., Lim, L., Ng, T., Lee, T., Mahendran, R., & Fones, C. (2004). The Prevalence of Psychiatric Disorders in Singapore Adults. *Annals Academy of Medicine Singapore, 33*(Suppl 5), S102.

Cocozza, J., & Skowyra, K. (2000). Youth with Mental Health Disorders: Issues and Emerging Responses. *Office of Juvenile Justice and Delinquency Prevention Journal, 7(1),* 3–13.

Dadds, M. R., Holland, D. E., Laurens, K. R., Mullins, M., Barrett, P. M., & Spence, S. H. (1999). Early intervention and prevention of anxiety disorders in children: Results at 2-year follow-up. *Journal of Consulting and Clinical Psychology, 67*(1), 145.

Engel, G. L. (1980). The clinical application of the biopsychosocial model. *The American Journal of Psychiatry.*

Fones, C., Kua, E., Ng, T., & Ko, S. (1998). Studying the mental health of a nation — A preliminary report on a population survey in Singapore. *Singapore Medical Journal, 39,* 251–255.

Fung, D. S. S., & Cai., Y. M. (2000). *Raise Your Child Right: A parenting guide for the 0–6 years old.* Singapore: Times Books International.

Fung, D. S. S., & Cai., Y. M. (Eds.). (2008). *A Primer of Child and Adolescent Psychiatry.* Singapore: World Scientific.

Grisso, T. (1999). Juvenile offenders and mental illness. *Psychiatry, Psychology and Law, 6*(2), 143–151.

Harrington, R., & Clark, A. (1998). Prevention and early intervention for depression in adolescence and early adult life. *European Archives of Psychiatry and Clinical Neuroscience, 248*(1), 32–45.

Hirshfeld-Becker, D. R., & Biederman, J. (2002). Rationale and principles for early intervention with young children at risk for anxiety disorders. *Clinical Child and Family Psychology Review, 5*(3), 161–172.

Hoe, Y. N. (2010, July, 26). Increase in suicide rates in S'pore, male suicides double that of female. *Channel News Asia.* Retrieved from http://www.channelnewsasia.com/stories/singaporelocalnews/view/1071583/1/.html

Kaiser, A. P., & Hester, P. P. (1997). Prevention of conduct disorder through early intervention: A social-communicative perspective. *Behavioral Disorders, 22*(3), 117–130.

Kessler, R., Amminger, G., Aguilar-Gaxiola, S., Alonso, J., Lee, S., & Ustün, T. (2007a). Age of onset of mental disorders: A review of recent literature. *Current opinion in psychiatry, 20*(4), 359.

Kessler, R., Angermeyer, M., Anthony, J., De Graaf, R., Demyttenaere, K., Gasquet, I., ... Ustun, T. (2007b). Lifetime prevalence and age-of-onset distributions of mental disorders in the World Health Organization's World Mental Health Survey Initiative. *World Psychiatry, 6*(3), 168–176.

Kessler, R., & Ustun, T. (2004). The world mental health (WMH) survey initiative version of the world health organization (WHO) composite international diagnostic interview (CIDI). *International Journal of Methods in Psychiatric Research, 13*(2), 93–121.

Liu, X., Kurita, H., Guo, C., Miyake, Y., Ze, J., & Cao, H. (1999). Prevalence and risk factors of behavioral and emotional problems among Chinese children aged 6 through 11 years. *Journal of the American Academy of Child & Adolescent Psychiatry, 38*(6), 708–715.

Ministry of Health. (2007, September 23). Strategic roadmap to build up a mentally resilient society [Press release]. Retrieved from http://www.moh.gov.sg/content/moh_web/home/pressRoom/pressRoomItemRelease/2007/strategic_roadmap_to_build_up_a_mentally_resilient_society.html

Ministry of Health. (2010). *Healthy Minds, Healthy Communities. National Mental Health Blueprint 2007–2012.* Retrieved from http://www.imh.com.sg/uploadedFiles/Publications/IMH%20National%20Mental%20Health%20Blueprint.pdf

Ministry of Health. (2011). Achieving more with less — Singapore's healthcare expenditure. Retrieved from http://www.moh.gov.sg/content/moh_web/home/Publications/educational_resources/2011/achieving_more_withless-singaporeshealthcareexpenditure.html

Ministry of Health. (2012). Singapore Healthcare System. Retrieved from http://www.moh.gov.sg/content/moh_web/home/our_healthcare_system.html

Murray, C. (1996). Rethinking DALYs. In C. J. L. Murray & A. D. Lopez, (Eds.), *The global burden of disease* (pp.1–98). Cambridge, Mass.: Harvard University Press.

National Healthcare Group (2011, November 18). *Latest study sheds light on the state of mental health in Singapore* [Press release]. Retrieved from http://www.nhg.com.sg/nhg_01_pressRelease2011_18Nov.asp?pr=2011

Ng, B. Y. (2001). *Till the break of day: a history of mental health services in Singapore, 1841–1993*: Singapore University Press.

Reach (2012). Oxford Dictionaries. Retrieved from http://oxforddictionaries.com/definition/reach?q=reach

Petersen, A. C., Compas, B. E., Brooks-Gunn, J., Stemmler, M., Ey, S., & Grant, K. E. (1993). Depression in adolescence. *American Psychologist, 48*(2), 155.

Phoon, W. (1972). Developing sound minds in healthy bodies. *Singapore Medical Journal, 13*(3), 119–125.

Phua, H., Chua, A., Ma, S., Heng, D., & Chew, S. (2009). Singapore's burden of disease and injury. *Singapore Medical Journal, 50*(5), 468–478.

Rappaport, G., Ornoy, A., & Tenenbaum, A. (1998). Is early intervention effective in preventing ADHD? *The Israel journal of psychiatry and related sciences, 35*(4), 271.

Robertson, A. A., Dill, P. L., Husain, J., & Undesser, C. (2004). Prevalence of mental illness and substance abuse disorders among incarcerated juvenile offenders in Mississippi. *Child Psychiatry & Human Development, 35*(1), 55–74.

Samaritans of Singapore. (2010). Suicide Statistics in Singapore — National Statistics 2010. Retrieved from http://www.samaritans.org.sg/suicide/stats.htm

Sawyer, M. G., Arney, F. M., Baghurst, P. A., Clark, J. J., Graetz, B. W., Kosky, R. J.,… Zubrick, S. R. (2001). The mental health of young people in Australia: key findings from the child and adolescent component of the national survey of mental health and well-being. *Australian and New Zealand Journal of Psychiatry, 35*(6), 806–814.

Srinath, S., Girimaji, S. C., Gururaj, G., Seshadri, S., Subbakrishna, D., Bhola, P., & Kumar N. (2005). Epidemiological study of child & adolescent psychiatric disorders in urban & rural areas of Bangalore, India. *Indian Journal of Medical Research, 122*(1), 67–79.

Tucci, J. (2004). The Singapore health system — Achieving positive health outcomes with low expenditure. *Healthcare Market Review, 26*.

U.S. Department of Education. (2001). *Twenty-third annual report to Congress on the implementation of the Individuals with Disabilities Education Act*. Washington, DC: Author.

Woo, B. S. C., Ng, T. P., Fung, D. S. S, Chan, Y. H., Lee, Y. P., Koh, J. B. K., & Cai, Y. M. (2007). Emotional and behavioural problems in Singaporean children based on parent, teacher and child reports. *Singapore Medical Journal, 48*(12), 1100–1106.

World Health Organization. (1992). *The ICD-10 classification of mental and behavioural disorders: Clinical descriptions and diagnostic guidelines.* Geneva, Switzerland: Author

World Health Organization (2008). *The Global Burden of Disease: 2004 Update.* Geneva, Switzerland: Author.

Chapter 1

Asia Australia Mental Health. (2011). *Asia — pacific community mental health development project — Summary report 2011 partnerships.* Retrieved from http://www.aamh.edu.au/special_projects/asia_pacific_community_mental_health_development_project

Bond, L., Patton. G., Glover, S., Carlin, J.B., Butler, H., Thomas, L., & Bowes, G. (2004). The gatehouse project: Can a multilevel school intervention affect emotional wellbeing and health risk behaviours? *Journal of Epidemiology Community Health, 58,* 997–1003.

Institute of Mental Health. (2012). Mental wellness. *Understanding your mental health.* Retrieved from http://www.imh.com.sg/wellness/page.aspx?id=356

Woo, B. S. C., Ng, T. P., Fung, D. S. S, Chan, Y. H., Lee, Y. P., Koh, J. B. K., & Cai, Y. M. (2007). Emotional and behavioural problems in Singaporean children based on parent, teacher and child reports. *Singapore Medical Journal, 48*(12), 1100–1106.

World Health Organization. (1995). *The health promoting school — A framework for action in the WHO western pacific region.* Manila: Regional Office for the Western Pacific, Author.

Chapter 2

Fung, D. S. S., Chua H. C., & Wong K. E. (2011). Singapore: Response, Early Assessment and Intervention in Community mental health. In Asia-Australia Mental Health, *A Community Partnership in Asia Pacific Community Mental Health Development Project Partnerships - Summary report 2011 (pp 79–84).* Retrieved from http://www.aamh.edu.au/special_projects/asia_pacific_community_mental_health_development_project

Fung D. S. S., & Lim-Ashworth, S. J. N. (2012). Opening minds: The use of technology to provide a personalized population based mental health programme. *Asia Pacific Biotech News, 16*(2), 35-37.

Institute of Mental Health. (2011, October 6). Mental health support for Special Education Schools [Press Release]. Retrieved from http://www.imh.com.sg/uploadedFiles/Newsroom/News_Releases/SPED%20news%20release.pdf

Ooi Y. P., Ang, R. P., Ibrahim, N. H., Koh, D., Lee, P. Y., Ong, L. P., Wong, G., & Fung, D. S. S. (in press). *The Continued Development and Practice of School Psychology in Singapore: Using REACH as an Illustration. School Psychology International.*

Chapter 3

Carvill, S. (2001). Sensory impairments, intellectual disability and psychiatry. *Journal of Intellectual Disability Research. Special Issue: Mental health and intellectual disability, 45(6)*, 467–483.

Dekker, M. C., & Koot, H. M. (2003). DSM-IV disorders in children with borderline to moderate intellectual disability. I: Prevalence and Impact. *Journal of the American Academy of Child & Adolescent Psychiatry. 42(8)*, 915–922.

Goodman, R. (1997). The strengths and difficulties questionnaire: A research note. *Journal of Child Psychology and Psychiatry, 38*, 581–586.

Guy, W. (1976). *ECDEU Assessment Manual for Psychopharmacology*. Rockville, MD: US Department of Health, Education, and Welfare Public Health Service Alcohol, Drug Abuse, and Mental Health Administration.

Hendren, R., Weisen, R.B., & Orley, J. (1994). *Mental health programmes in schools*. Retrieved from http://whqlibdoc.who.int/hq/1993/WHO_MNH_PSF_93.3_Rev.1.pdf

Koh, D., & Boon, J. (2012). *Evaluation of a community-based mental health service for children and youths in Singapore: Looking at the Response Early intervention and Assessment for Community Mental Health (REACH) Programme*. Manuscript in preparation.

Koh, D., Sulaiman, R., Ooi, Y. P., & Fung, D. (2011). Clinical outcomes of a community mental health programme for youths. *Singapore Annals of the Academy of Medicine, 40 (11)*, S43.

Ministry of Education. (2012a). *Compulsory education*. Retrieved from http://www.moe.gov.sg/initiatives/compulsory-education/

Ministry of Education. (2012b). *School information service: School clusters and cluster super-intendents*. Retrieved from http://app.sis.moe.gov.sg/schinfo/schoolclusters.asp

Ministry of Education. (2012c). *Allied educator counselling*. Retrieved from http://www.moe.gov.sg/careers/allied-educators/counselling/

Noterdaeme, M. A., & Wriedt, E. (2010). Comorbidity in autism spectrum disorders — I: Mental retardation and psychiatric comorbidity. *Zeitschrift für Kinder- und Jugendpsychiatrie und Psychotherapie, 38(4)*, 257–266.

Soo, G., Ong, J. G. X., Chen, A., & Ong, L. P. (2011). Mental health literacy of Singapore school counsellors: A preliminary study. *Annuals of the Academy of Medicine, Singapore, 40 (11)*, S214.

Sulaiman, S. R., Ong, L. P., & Fung, D. (2009, October 16–17). Preliminary evidence for the effectiveness of the REACH community mental health programme. Poster presented at the National Healthcare Group Annual Scientific Congress. Singapore.

Taggart, L., Cousins, W., & Milner, S. (2007). Young people with learning disabilities living in state care: Their emotional, behavioural and mental health status. *Child Care in Practice. Special Issue: Going from strength to strength-promoting children's mental health, 13(4)*, 401–416.

The EuroQol Group. (1990). EuroQol-a new facility for the measurement of health related quality of life. *Health Policy, 16(3)*, 199–208.

World Health Organization. (2005). *Mental health policy and service guidance package : Child and adolescent mental health policies and plans.* Geneva: Author. Retrieved from http://www.who.int/mental_health/policy/Childado_mh_module.pdf

World Health Organization. (2003). *Mental health policy and service packages: Organization of services for mental health.* Geneva: Author. Retrieved from http://www.who.int/mental_health/resources/en/Organization.pdf

Chapter 4

Thornicroft, G., & Tansella, M. (2003). What are the arguments for community-based mental health care? *Copenhagen, WHO Regional Office for Europe (Health Evidence Network report.* Retrieved from http://www.euro.who.int/document/E82976.pdf

Tyrer, P., Coid, J., Simmonds, S., Joseph, P., & Marriott, S. (1999). Community mental health team management for those with severe mental illnesses and disordered

VWO partners

About VWOs, Charities and IPCs
http://www.ncss.org.sg/vwocorner/about_vwo.asp

Chapter 5

Institute of Mental Health. (2011, July 12). GPs go back to school to beef up mental health expertise [Press Release]. Retrieved from http://www.imh.com.sg/uploadedFiles/Newsroom/News_Releases/12Jul10_GPs%20to%20beef%20up%20mental%20health%20expertise.pdf

Ministry of Health. (2012). Healthcare Institution Statistics. Retrieved from http://www.moh.gov.sg/content/moh_web/home/statistics/healthcare_institutionstatistics.html

Ministry of Health. (2010). *Healthy Minds, Healthy Communities. National Mental Health Blueprint 2007–2012.* Retrieved from http://www.imh.com.sg/uploadedFiles/Publications/IMH%20National%20Mental%20Health%20Blueprint.pdf

World Health Organization. (2005). *Mental health policy and service guidance package : Child and adolescent mental health policies and plans.* Geneva: Author. Retrieved from http://www.who.int/mental_health/policy/Childado_mh_module.pdf

Chapter 6

Albano, A. M., & Kendall, P. C. (2002). Cognitive behavioural therapy for children and adolescents with anxiety disorders: Clinical research advances. *International Review of Psychiatry, 14,* 129–134.

American Psychiatric Association (2000) *Diagnostic and statistical manual of mental disorders* (4th ed., text revision). Washington, DC: Author.

Ang, R. P., & Fung, D. S. S. (2006). *Seeing Red: Help your child deal with anger at home and in public.* Singapore: SNP International.

Ang, R. P., & Ooi, Y. P. (2003). *Helping angry children and youth: Strategies that work. Training manual.* Singapore: Armour Publishing.

Anstendig, K. D. (1999). Is selective mutism an anxiety disorder? Rethinking its DSM-IV classification. *Journal Anxiety Disorder, 13,* 417–34.

Black, B., & Uhde, T. W. (1995). Psychiatric characteristics of children with selective mutism: a pilot study. *Journal of American Academy Child Adolescent Psychiatry 34,* 847–56.

Dunn, W., & Bennett, D. (2002). Patterns of sensory processing in children with attention deficit hyperactivity disorder. *The Occupational Therapy Journal of Research, 22(1),* 4–15.

Flannery-Schroeder, E. C., & Kendall, P. C. (2000). Group and individual cognitive-behavioral treatments for youth with anxiety-disorders: A randomized clinical trial. *Cognitive Therapy and Research, 24(3),* 251–278.

Fung, D. S. S., Manassis, K., Kenny, A., & Fiksenbaum, L. (2002). Web-based CBT for selective mutism. *Journal of American Academy Child Adolescent Psychiatry, 41,* 112–3.

Kendall, P. C. (1994). Treating anxiety disorders in children: results of a randomised clinical trial. *Journal of Consulting and Clinical Psychology, 62,* 100–10.

Mangeot, S.D., Miller, L.J. McIntosh, D.N., McGrath-Clarke, J. Simon, J., Hagerman, R. J., & Goldson E. (2001). Sensory modulation dysfunction in children with attention deficit hyperactivity disorder. *Developmental Medicine and Child Neurology, 43,* 399–406.

Mythily, S., Qiu, S., & Winslow, M. (2008). Prevalence and correlates of excessive internet use among youth in Singapore. *Annals Academy of Medicine Singapore, 37,* 9–14.

Parush, S., Suhmer, H., Steinberg, A., & Kaitz, M. (1997). Somatosensory functioning in children with attention deficit hyperactivity disorder. *Developmental Medicine and Child Neurology, 39,* 464–468.

Smith-Roley, S., Blanche, E.I., & Schaaf, R.C. (2001). *Understanding the nature of sensory integration with diverse population.* San Antonio, TX: Therapy Skill Builders.

Chapter 7

Chan , W. (2010, November 8). 1 in 10 children aged 6–16 has mental health disorders: IMH expert. *New Straits Times.* Retrieved from http://www.channelnewsasia.com/stories/singaporelocalnews/view/1092048/1/.hml

Koh, D., Sulaiman, R., Ooi, Y. P., & Fung, D. S. S. (2011). Clinical Outcomes of a Community Mental Health Programme for Youths in Singapore. *Annals of the Academy of Medicine, Singapore, 40 (11)*, S43.

Sulaiman, S. R., Ong, L. P., & Fung, D. S. S. (2009). Preliminary Evidence for the Effectiveness of the REACH Community Mental Health Programme. Poster Presented during the National Healthcare Group Annual Scientific Congress., October 16–17, 2009.

Glossary

American Psychiatric Association (APA). (2000). *Diagnostic and Statistical Manual of Mental Disorders — Fourth Edition Text Revision (DSM-IV TR)*. Washington, DC: American Psychiatric Association.

World Health Organization (WHO). (2007). *What is mental health?* Retrieved from:http://www.who.int/features/qa/62/en/index.html

World Health Organization (WHO). (2010). *International Statistical Classification of Diseases and Related Health Problems Tenth Revision*. Geneva: Author.

www.ingramcontent.com/pod-product-compliance
Lightning Source LLC
Chambersburg PA
CBHW070339270326
41926CB00017B/3922